THE HIGH-PROTEIN BARIATRIC COOKBOOK

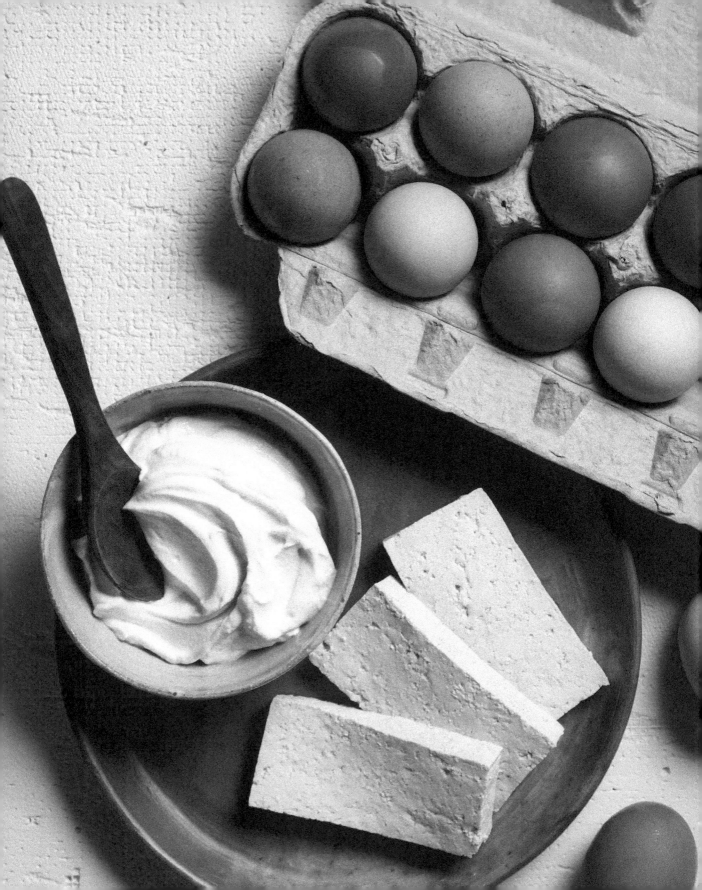

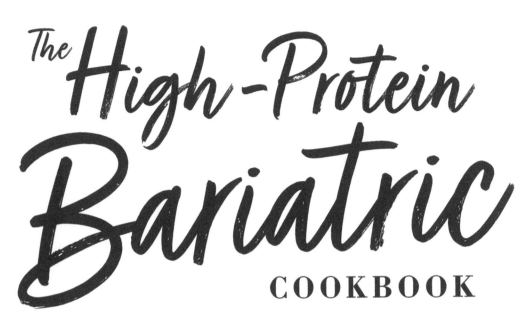

The High-Protein Bariatric COOKBOOK

ESSENTIAL RECIPES FOR RECOVERY AND LIFELONG WEIGHT MANAGEMENT

Staci Gulbin, MS, MEd, RD

Photography by Tara Donne

ROCKRIDGE PRESS

Interior and Cover Designer: Brian Lewis
Photo Art Director/Art Manager: Samantha Ulban
Editor: Rachelle Cihonski
Production Editor: Ashley Polikoff
Photography © Tara Donne. Food Styling by Cyd McDowell.

Cover: Fish Taco Bowl with Cauliflower Rice, p.93.

ISBN: Print 978-1-64739-778-4
eBook 978-1-64739-464-6

R0

This book is dedicated to all my clients over the years who inspired me to help others create a healthier life for themselves.

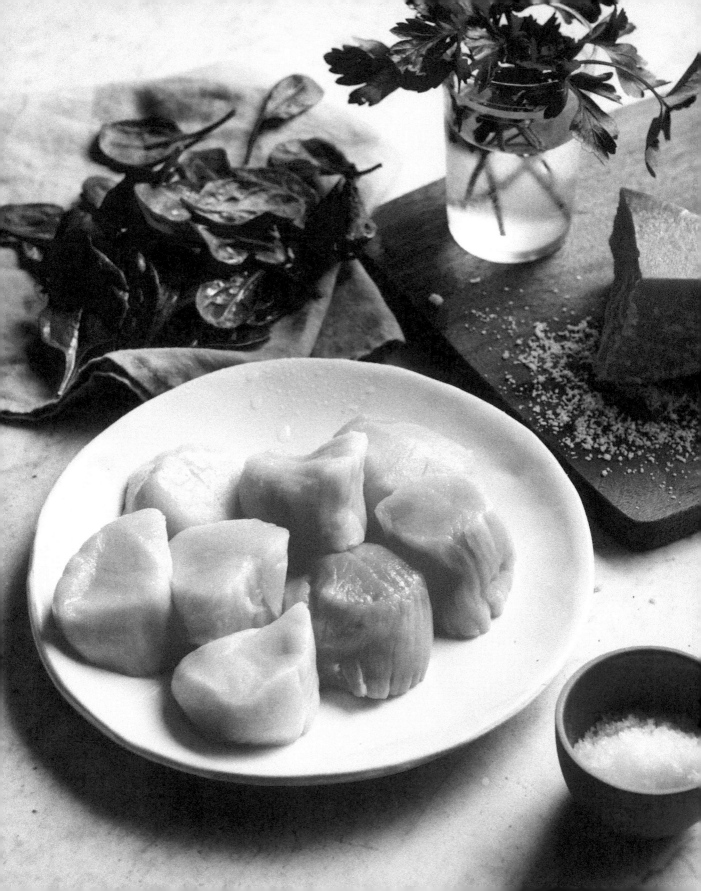

CONTENTS

INTRODUCTION

Welcome! If you're reading this book, it means you're ready to give healthy eating after bariatric surgery your absolute best effort. And for that you should be immensely proud of yourself.

Healthy eating after bariatric surgery is not easy. I know this because I have a decade of experience as a registered dietitian, and several of those years have been spent working with bariatric surgery patients.

I was there from the day patients started their pre-op phase, including meeting their weight loss goals to gain approval for surgery, through the various stages of post-op as they faced struggles with textured foods, pain, or discomfort, as well as through their successes and growing confidence.

The pre-op phase before bariatric surgery can, in and of itself, seem like a strenuous exercise. But if you look at it as the beginning of a new chapter and open your mind to the changes ahead, then the time will fly by. Before you know it, you will be looking toward your surgery date.

There are, of course, new hurdles to overcome once you have surgery, but just as the chapters in this book appear one at a time, you should look at the post-bariatric surgery phases one at a time, one day at a time. Along the way, be open to help from others, listen to the advice of those health professionals caring for you, and be forgiving of yourself if everything doesn't go as planned.

It's in those unplanned moments, good or bad, when you can learn and grow the most. Believe me when I tell you that your bariatric surgery journey will have ups and downs, but there are many wonderful things you can look forward to.

Patients would enter my office post-op with a smile on their face so big it would light up the room after they told me they could buckle their seatbelt without an extender. Or they would be excited to tell me they can now ride amusement rides with their children or walk in the park without getting out of breath. The most common first non-scale victory that they would mention is the increased energy they have within the first month after surgery.

This book will take you through each step of your bariatric journey, from what to expect to eat pre-op to your nutritional goals post-op. You will learn how much of the major nutrients your body will need for optimal health, as well as the tools and resources that will help you be successful.

And if you're worried you won't be able to prepare the recipes in this book, no need to worry. I know people of all cooking experience levels will be reading this book, so I have made the recipes easy to follow without requiring numerous ingredients.

I am confident that after reading this book, you will feel more excited than ever to tackle your bariatric surgery journey. You will learn that eating healthy can be delicious and that you can still enjoy your favorite foods in a healthier way.

As you create each recipe, you will become better at cooking and will gain confidence in meal preparation. This skill will help you maintain your health for years to come and will allow you to teach others how to be healthy, too.

You can do this! I have faith in you. I'm excited for your journey and for the successes you will encounter along the way. And I look forward to your reading the pages to come and enjoying each recipe. This is just the beginning of a new chapter for you and for your health. Enjoy!

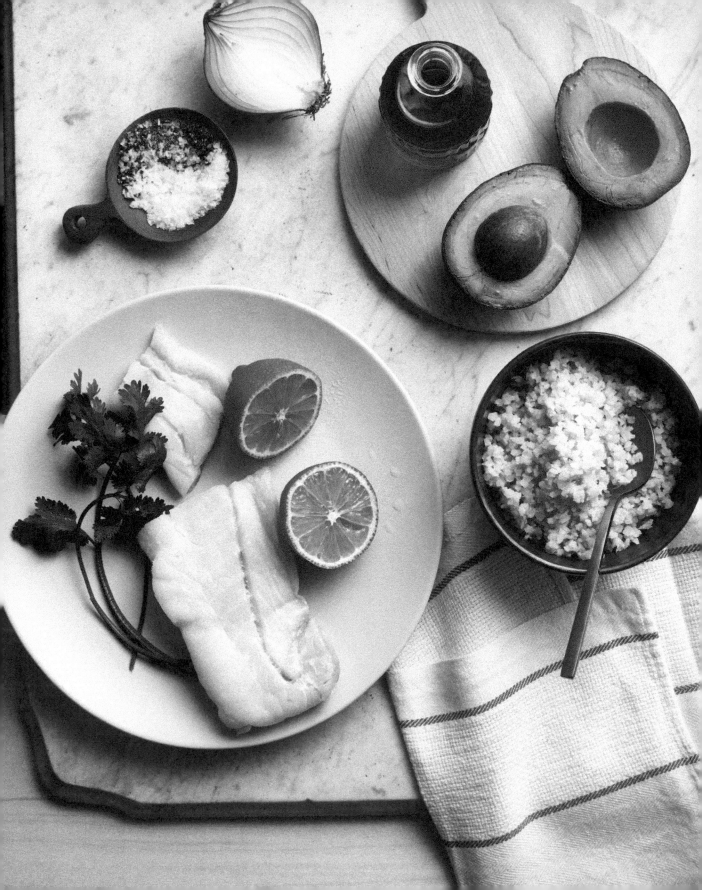

CHAPTER ONE

A Healthier, Empowered You

This is not your average post-op bariatric surgery cookbook. Along with plenty of delicious protein-packed recipes in the pages to come, in this chapter, you'll find helpful information about what your diet will look like in the initial stages after surgery. Once you've graduated from the various textured phases of post-op, we'll discuss what eating will look like beyond the first three months, including what nutrients you'll need daily to maintain weight loss and overall health.

To ensure long-term success, this chapter will also explain how to make small lifestyle changes outside of eating that are vital to keeping the weight off and staying healthy in body and mind.

YOUR NEW RELATIONSHIP WITH FOOD

From the moment you considered undergoing bariatric surgery, your relationship with food likely started to evolve. The way you think about and feel around food will continue to change throughout this post-op journey and for years to come.

You may have already started making a lot of changes to your diet just to qualify for surgery. The thought of making more changes may take away any enjoyment from mealtime, or maybe the thought of having to prepare different textures of food sounds stressful. If you're not experienced in cooking, you may worry you won't be able to follow the guidelines in each post-op stage.

Just remember that in most cases, you'll have your healthcare team available for support and guidance throughout your journey. What's more, this book will provide you with the basics of what you'll need for success. It's not going to be easy, and it's not going to happen overnight, but it will be a learning experience through which you will grow toward better health.

Pre-Op Dieting

If you haven't yet undergone surgery, your doctor may have advised you to lose some weight. There are some general guidelines you can follow to increase your chances for weight loss during this pre-op phase.

Not everyone will lose weight pre-op or will need to lose weight. What's important at this stage is to learn which nutrients your body will need after surgery for long-term health. Also, you should try new foods, prepare foods in new ways, and eat smaller portion sizes at mealtime to prepare for post-op life.

Below is an example of what you should eat in a pre-op day to help you prepare for post-op.

Breakfast: 8 to 12 ounces of unsweetened almond milk or water mixed with 1 to 2 scoops of sugar-free or low-sugar whey protein shake (less than 5 grams of carbohydrates per scoop)

CONTINUES »

Morning Snack: 8 to 12 ounces of unsweetened almond milk or water mixed with 1 to 2 scoops of sugar-free or low-sugar whey protein shake (less than 5 grams of carbohydrates per scoop) OR an 11-ounce commercially prepared protein shake (less than 10 grams of sugar)

Lunch: 2 hard-boiled eggs

Afternoon Snack: 1 cup nonstarchy vegetables like raw broccoli with 2 tablespoons low-sugar Greek yogurt dressing

Dinner: 4 ounces grilled chicken breast, 2 cups steamed green beans, 2 tablespoons light margarine

Even though the recipes in this book are primarily geared toward losing weight and staying healthy after surgery, you can also use these recipes pre-op for the same purpose. All the recipes in this book contain more grams of protein than carbohydrate per serving and provide guidelines for portion sizes.

ONE STEP AT A TIME

Bariatric surgery is a brave undertaking that may leave you feeling overwhelmed. That's why it's important to take things one step at a time. Below are five important steps for success in your post-op journey.

1. **Learn about the diet.** Your doctor will likely provide you with informational documents about the post-op bariatric surgery diet before you even have surgery. However, these instructions may be just another worksheet to add to your growing pile. It may help to organize these papers into a binder in categories by stage. Take about 15 minutes each day to read through the stage of the diet you're on so you understand it.

2. **Prepare your home to make post-op life easy.** Because you'll likely be recovering from post-op at home, it's important to have your kitchen organized to make post-op success easy. First, dedicate a cabinet or pantry shelf as well as a shelf in your refrigerator for your post-op food. This will make your food accessible and will help you see when you're running low. Second, keep a running list hung up where you can easily see it. As you run out of a staple food or drink item, write it down on your list so you can grab it on your next shopping trip.

3. **Create your post-op meal plan.** If possible, start creating your post-op plan before your surgery date. Have a list of acceptable meals ready for the first few stages of your diet. Before you graduate from each texture, start planning your next stage so you can create a grocery list for when the time comes. Also, learn as much as you can about protein to help make meeting your protein goals after surgery easier.

4. **Prep your meals.** In the first two post-op stages (liquid and puree) prep will be fairly quick, taking about an hour each week. For the later stages of the diet, prep may take a bit longer, but having foods ready and available will ensure you stick to your healthy regimen.

5. **Start your food journal.** A food journal will be a vital part of your post-op journey. You can write down or type in everything you eat during the day, including portion sizes, and how much water you drink. Also, tracking symptoms can remind you of foods that your body may not be able to tolerate well after surgery. You can then avoid these foods and report such findings to your medical team.

Protein: The Most Important Nutrient

Although carbohydrates and fats are important to overall health, protein is an especially important macronutrient during your bariatric journey. Consuming protein can help:

- **Assist in wound healing.** Protein is needed for the body to repair muscle, skin, and other tissues, as well as deliver oxygen to tissues throughout the body.

- **Support metabolism.** After bariatric surgery, especially during the early periods of rapid weight loss, you'll be at risk for losing lean muscle mass. This can have a negative impact on your recovery, strength, mobility, and metabolic health long-term.

- **Keep you fuller longer.** Because it takes your body longer to digest protein than carbohydrates, it will help keep you fuller longer.

- **Form important compounds in the body.** Protein helps in the production of hormones, enzymes, and immune system antibodies that help the body function properly. Without enough protein, the immune system can weaken and in turn will negatively impact other areas of health.

CONTINUES »

When it comes to types of protein, they are not all created equal. There are three major types of proteins.

- **Complete proteins** contain adequate levels of all the essential amino acids needed for optimal health and work more efficiently in muscle-building processes in the body. Foods that contain complete proteins include soybeans, milk, whey protein, beef, eggs, and other animal-based foods.

- **Incomplete proteins** do not contain enough of each of the nine essential amino acids. These include legumes, cereals, vegetables, nuts, seeds, and seaweed.

- **Complementary proteins** fill in the gaps when it comes to essential amino acids. If a certain food is missing an amino acid or doesn't contain enough of a certain amino acid, it can be paired with another food that contains it so that the pair can make a complete protein. Examples of complementary proteins include grains and beans or legumes, such as rice and beans. The foods do not have to be eaten at the same meal if they are eaten in the same day.

CHOOSING YOUR PROTEIN

When it comes to post-op eating, choose foods that have a high protein-to-calorie ratio. In the first three months post-op, you will only be able to tolerate small portions of food and will be consuming less than 1000 calories daily. Therefore, you must make the most of every calorie you consume, with protein being the priority.

A simple rule of thumb is to consume at least 10 grams of protein for every 100 calories. The lower the calories per gram of protein, the better off you will be.

FOOD	AMOUNT	CALORIES	PROTEIN (GRAMS)	QUALITY
Whey protein powder, sugar-free	1 tablespoon	90	20	High
Chicken breast	1 ounce	47	9	High
Albacore tuna fish, flaked	1 ounce	25	5.5	High
Greek yogurt, plain, unsweetened	½ cup	60	12	High

CONTINUES »

FOOD	AMOUNT	CALORIES	PROTEIN (GRAMS)	QUALITY
Cottage cheese, low-fat	½ cup	82	14	High
Mozzarella cheese, part-skim, low-fat	1 ounce	78	8	High
Tofu	1 ounce	21	2	High
Atlantic salmon	1 ounce	59	5.6	Moderate-High
Egg	1 large	70	6	Moderate-High
Black beans	1 ounce	25	2	Moderate
Cow's milk, low-fat	½ cup	52	4	Moderate
Plain, unsweetened soymilk	½ cup	40	3.5	Moderate
Ground beef, lean	1 ounce	93	4	Low
Peanut butter	1 tablespoon	95	4	Low
Chia seeds	1 tablespoon	69	2.35	Low

A NOTE ON PLANT-BASED PROTEINS

Whether you follow a meatless diet or just wish to eat less meat, there are plenty of plant-based protein options, including beans and lentils, edamame, nutritional yeast, tempeh and tofu, and nuts. Some plant-based proteins are not as bioavailable as animal proteins, which means they have a lower impact on muscle-building in the body.

Furthermore, certain nutrients found primarily in animal-based proteins, like vitamin B_{12}, must be taken in supplement form by those who follow a meatless diet. This is because forms of vitamin B_{12} in plant-based proteins like seaweed are not reliable sources. The only trusted sources of vitamin B_{12} in a meatless diet are fortified plant-based milks and cereals, as well as vitamin B_{12} supplements. If you follow a meatless diet, it's important to visit the doctor regularly to have your iron, vitamin B_{12}, and vitamin D levels checked so you can ensure that you're consuming and absorbing enough of these nutrients daily.

THE FIRST THREE MONTHS

The first three months after bariatric surgery will set the stage for your post-op journey. It's a challenging time, but exciting, too, since you'll be learning how your newly configured stomach works. Your journey may look different from others', because your diet progression will be determined by your individual bariatric team. The timelines listed below provide a typical schedule that most will follow. Feel free to adjust the timelines according to how your body is healing and how long it takes for your new stomach to become used to digesting foods again.

Lapband
First 1 to 2 Days: Clear liquids
Weeks 1 to 2: Liquids
Week 3: Pureed foods
Weeks 4 to 6: Soft foods
Weeks 7 to 8+: General diet

Gastric Sleeve
First 1 to 2 Days: Clear liquids
Weeks 1 to 2: Liquids
Week 3: Pureed foods
Week 4: Soft foods
Weeks 5 to 6+: General diet

What to Avoid

The following is a list of foods you will need to avoid in the first three months.

- **Foods high in sugar:** Aim for foods with no more than 15 grams of sugar per serving.
- **Fatty and fried foods:** French fries, cream-based sauces and soups, premium ice cream, whipped cream, fried chicken, and other fried foods will not be tolerated well in your new stomach.
- **"Empty" calories that don't contain a good source of protein, vitamins, or minerals:** Salty snacks like chips, sugary colas and juices, candy, and baked goods should be avoided post-op.

- **Raw fruits and vegetables:** Although vegetables are good for you, your body will not tolerate raw fruits and vegetables well in the first three months after surgery.
- **Bread, rice, and pasta:** Starchy foods are typically low in protein and will expand in your stomach when you eat them. In other words, they will take up a lot of real estate in your stomach without providing much protein or nutrient value.
- **Caffeine and alcohol:** Caffeine can irritate the stomach lining and, in turn, increase the risk of ulcers. Alcohol and many caffeinated beverages typically contain high amounts of carbohydrates and calories that are not beneficial to weight loss, not to mention that alcohol metabolism in your body will be altered post-op. This means drinking alcohol, even in small amounts, can impact your body more than it did before surgery, so limit it to reduce risk of harmful health issues.

If you consume foods that you should avoid, you may experience symptoms like abdominal cramping, diarrhea, nausea, vomiting, gas, bloating, and swelling. If you experience such symptoms, contact your healthcare team right away so they can help determine what caused them and how to prevent them from reoccurring.

Liquids

The liquid phase after bariatric surgery comes in two steps: clear liquid and full liquid. The clear liquid phase occurs while you're still in the hospital and includes broth, sugar-free gelatin, water, and perhaps sugar-free ice pops. You'll be on this diet until you tolerate the clear liquids well without any symptoms.

The full liquid diet, which starts one to three days after surgery, will last about two weeks and is a time when you should consume plenty of protein to help maintain your lean muscle mass, as well as support post-op healing and healthy metabolism. Examples of foods and beverages acceptable on the full liquid diet include:

- Low-sugar protein shakes
- Strained low-fat creamy soups
- Skim milk with protein powder
- Nonfat, unsweetened plain yogurt
- Low-fat or nonfat cottage cheese

- ◆ Ricotta cheese made with skim milk
- ◆ Sugar-free juices, gelatin, puddings, and ice pops
- ◆ Decaffeinated tea and coffee

DAILY NUTRITIONAL GOALS

Protein: 50 to 70 grams

Calories: 300 to 600

Number of meals: 5 to 8 small meals

Fluids: at least 48 to 64 ounces

Vitamins and supplements: multivitamin, calcium (at least 1200 milligrams/day), vitamin D (about 1000 International Units/day), vitamin B_{12} (500 to 1000 micrograms/day); you may need to take other supplements daily as recommended by your doctor

SAMPLE DAY MEAL PLAN

Breakfast: Peaches and Creamy Coconut Smoothie (page 28)

Morning Snack: 1 cup low-fat cottage cheese

Lunch: Lemon Meringue Pie Smoothie (page 30)

Afternoon Snack: Savory Beef Bone Broth (page 24)

Dinner: Commercial protein shake (about 11 ounces) with at least 20 grams of protein

WHAT TO AVOID

Spices may be irritating at this stage. Also, avoid carbonated drinks or chewing gum since they can allow air to enter the pouch of your stomach and can cause pain.

HEALTHY HABITS

No straws! This is a lifelong habit. Straws cause air to enter the pouch which is not only painful to pass, but also takes up space in your smaller stomach that could be used to house protein. Also, drink slowly with small sips during this phase and wait to drink fluids 30 minutes before or after eating anything.

Pureed Foods

At about the third week after surgery, if full liquids were tolerated well, you may start adding in pureed foods. Pureed foods are blended foods that are smooth in texture with no bumps or lumps. Examples of foods on this stage of the diet include:

- Unsweetened applesauce
- Well-cooked pureed vegetables
- Cooked cereals
- Mashed potatoes
- Scrambled eggs or egg substitute
- Canned fruit
- Strained or pureed meat or poultry
- Canned tuna fish
- Tofu
- Any foods from the full liquid or liquid stage

DAILY NUTRITIONAL GOALS

Protein: 50 to 70 grams
Calories: no more than 500
Number of meals: 5 to 8 small meals
Fluids: at least 64 ounces, or more if tolerated
Vitamins and supplements: multivitamin, calcium (at least 1200 milligrams/day), vitamin D (about 1000 International Units/day), vitamin B_{12} (500 to 1000 micrograms/day); you may need to take other supplements daily as recommended by your doctor

SAMPLE DAY MEAL PLAN

Breakfast: 1 cup low-fat cottage cheese and ½ cup unsweetened applesauce
Morning Snack: Harvest Vegetable Chicken Bone Broth (page 25)
Lunch: Broccoli-Cheddar Puree (page 37)
Afternoon Snack: Tuna-Avocado Salad (page 35)
Dinner: Commercial protein shake (about 11 ounces) with at least 20 grams of protein

WHAT TO AVOID

Any fibrous vegetables or hard textures will be difficult to digest. Remove any peels or seeds before cooking and eating.

| HEALTHY HABITS

Start using a small utensil, such as a child's spoon, to practice taking small bites while eating. This will help prevent you from eating too much in one bite, and in turn prevent uncomfortable symptoms.

Soft Foods

After the first month or two after surgery, you may graduate to the soft food phase. In this phase you can have anything you consumed in the earlier stages along with:

- Mashed cooked vegetables
- Ground meats like lean turkey or beef
- Steamed fish
- Beans or lentils

| DAILY NUTRITIONAL GOALS

Protein: 60 to 80 grams

Calories: no more than 1000

Number of meals: 6 small meals

Fluids: at least 64 ounces, or more if tolerated

Vitamins and supplements: multivitamin, calcium (at least 1200 milligrams/day), vitamin D (about 1000 International Units/day), vitamin B_{12} (500 to 1000 micrograms/day); you may need to take other supplements daily as recommended by your doctor

| SAMPLE DAY MEAL PLAN

Breakfast: Cinnamon-Spice Overnight Cereal (page 55)

Morning Snack: Cheesy Cauliflower Tots (page 146)

Lunch: Lemon-Dill Cod with Sautéed Veggie Salsa (page 91)

Afternoon Snack: Commercial protein shake (about 11 ounces) with at least 20 grams of protein)

Dinner: Crustless Turkey Pot Pie (page 114)

Evening Snack: Strawberry Gelatin Tea (page 151)

| WHAT TO AVOID

No steak or solid meats during this phase. Stick to ground meats and flaked fish.

Even though the food is soft, start practicing chewing your food well during this phase to assist digestion.

General Foods

Once you have successfully tolerated the foods in the soft foods phase of the diet, then you can graduate to a general foods diet. This phase is basically just normal-textured, healthy eating. You will still limit sugar, fat, and total carbohydrate during this phase, but may eat raw fruits and vegetables and solid meats as tolerated.

| DAILY NUTRITIONAL GOALS

Protein: 60 to 100 grams

Calories: about 1000, or more as recommended by your doctor

Number of meals: 6 small meals

Fluids: at least 64 ounces, or more if tolerated

Vitamins and supplements: multivitamin, calcium (at least 1200 milligrams/day), vitamin D (about 1000 International Units/day), vitamin B_{12} (500 to 1000 micrograms/day); you may need to take other supplements daily as recommended by your doctor

| SAMPLE DAY MEAL PLAN

Breakfast: Italian-Style Scramble (page 46)

Morning Snack: Cheesecake Cottage Cheese (page 52)

Lunch: Fish Taco Bowl with Cauliflower Rice (page 93)

Afternoon Snack: Garlic-Parmesan Cheesy Chips (page 142)

Dinner: Almond-Crusted Chicken Tenders (page 102)

Evening Snack: Commercial protein shake (about 11 ounces) with at least 20 grams of protein)

| WHAT TO AVOID

During this phase, you should be able to tolerate most food textures. Just avoid anything that you identify in your food and symptom diary as causing symptoms.

Once-a-week tracking can help you stay on board with your healthy habits and ensure you're consuming enough nutrients daily.

Drinking Your Protein

During your bariatric post-op journey, protein shakes are a convenient and low-calorie protein source.

What makes a good protein shake?

- **At least one high-quality source of protein:** This means either whey protein powder; a plant-based protein powder with at least 10 grams of protein per 100 calories (such as a pea protein powder product like Orgain); or plain, unsweetened nonfat Greek yogurt.

- **Fiber:** Fiber in your protein shake will help prevent constipation. Since you will not be able to eat raw vegetables or solid vegetables quite yet, it's important to consume fiber in some form during the first three months after surgery. Add in frozen low-carbohydrate fruits and vegetables like strawberries, blueberries, and baby spinach, or seeds like chia or flax for fiber.

- **Flavored extracts:** Extracts are a low- to no-calorie way to add flavor to your protein shakes. Look in the spices section of the grocery store or online for a variety of sugar-free syrups or extracts you can use without adding sugar or calories.

- **Proper ratios:** The basics of a protein shake include about 1 cup plain nonfat Greek yogurt or 1 cup milk mixed with 1 tablespoon protein powder and either ½ cup frozen fruit or 1 tablespoon nut butter. Then, for flavor add about 1 teaspoon of extract, cocoa powder, and/or flavored sugar-free syrup or low- to no-calorie sweetener.

You can buy a pre-made protein shake to save time or make your own. If you make your own protein shakes, the flavor profiles are limitless, and you will know the ingredients going in them. Then, when you have symptoms, it will be easier to identify what the possible cause may be. However, there may be times when a prepackaged protein shake will be more convenient, so do what works for you and helps you stick to your nutrition goals.

EATING WELL FOR LIFE

Once you're on the general foods diet, it may become tempting to fall into old eating habits, since you can tolerate most, if not all, textures. This is an exciting time since you will start to feel like you're eating "normally" again. However, it's important to remember that your stomach and digestive system are still different than they were before. You'll still have to follow a lower-carbohydrate, high-protein diet to maintain optimal health. Let's cover what your daily intake of each nutrient should look like.

Protein

Protein is going to be a vital part of your weight loss and maintenance success for life, so it's important that you continue to plan meals around protein and then include fiber-rich vegetables. You should consume 60 to 100 grams of protein daily, depending on your activity level and medical conditions.

Carbohydrates

You will have to follow a lower-carbohydrate diet for life after bariatric surgery. Research shows that staying around 130 grams of carbohydrate or less daily, or about 40 percent of your calories from carbohydrates, is best for long-term weight loss success. For example, if you consume 1200 calories daily, consume no more than 480 calories from carbohydrates. Since each gram of carbohydrate is about 4 calories, that comes out to about 120 grams of carbohydrates.

Fats

It's important to stick to a low-fat diet for life, since you will likely not tolerate fatty foods well. Therefore, trim fats from meats, choose ground meats that are at least 90 percent lean, and avoid any seafood products canned in oil. You should consume no more than 5 grams of fat per serving during meals. To reduce fat in your diet, use dry cooking methods like baking, grilling, roasting, or steaming, or pan-fry with healthy fats like olive oil. And if you do consume fats in your diet, choose healthy fats rich in omega-3 fatty acids, such as those found in avocado and salmon.

Hydration

Consume at least 64 ounces of low- to no-calorie fluid daily to stay hydrated. You may be able to drink more during each sip, but try to avoid gulping. Carbonated drinks may be allowed in small amounts, but check with your doctor first.

Vitamins and Mineral Supplements

You'll need to take vitamin and mineral supplements for the rest of your life, but the dosages may differ as you consume a more nutrient-dense diet. Check with your doctor to have your labs checked at least every year to see if your vitamin or mineral levels are low and adjust your dosage and/or diet as needed.

Your Plate After Bariatric Surgery

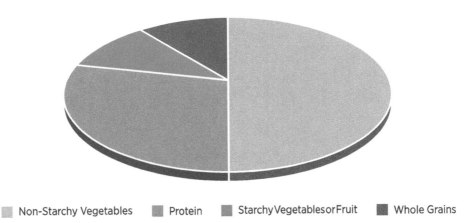

| Non-Starchy Vegetables | Protein | Starchy Vegetables or Fruit | Whole Grains |

This diagram shows what your plate should look like during your general diet phase. Most of your plate should be low-carbohydrate, nonstarchy vegetables and protein. Small portions of your plate should be used for starchy vegetables, fruit, or whole grains. Continue to limit fats during the general diet phase as they may not be tolerated well after surgery. Consume only healthy fats from sources like avocado, plant-based oils like olive oil, or fish rich in omega-3 fatty acids such as salmon or tuna.

All in Moderation with 80/20

Some bariatric experts use the 80/20 principle of eating to help coach bariatric patients. This way of eating means using 80 percent of your daily calories for consuming nutrient-dense foods, while eating the other 20 percent for pleasure. If you're eating 1000 calories a day, for example, then 200 of those calories can be discretionary calories.

Your discretionary calories in a post-op 80/20 bariatric diet may be used for foods like fruit other than berries; starchy foods like rice, pasta, or potatoes (if tolerated); low-sugar frozen yogurt; baked potato chips or pretzels (if tolerated); or sugar-free or low-sugar dark chocolate.

It's important to remember that you should not follow this type of regimen until you are on a general diet, at least 6 to 12 months after surgery. Before you start loosening your diet with this method, make sure you have been successful in complying with your healthy diet guidelines and have been losing weight post-op. If you're not sure if this is right for you, then talk with the registered dietitian on your surgical team.

SETTING UP YOUR KITCHEN

Preparation is everything when it comes to successful healthy eating. Making sure your kitchen has what you need is vital to success. Here are some basic steps you should take to prepare your kitchen for post-op living.

Clean out your pantry and refrigerator. If you have any high-carbohydrate foods or beverages in your kitchen, get rid of them. Donate unopened, nonperishable foods to your local food bank. For perishable foods that are unopened, give them to a friend or family member or throw them away to prevent any temptation. Don't try to consume any leftovers in a "last supper" type way, as this can make you feel sick and is not teaching you healthy eating habits. If you have other people in your house consuming such foods, simply place these foods in a separate shelf or cabinet.

Have healthy pantry staples on hand. It's important to have certain nonperishable ingredients on hand that will be helpful during your post-op bariatric diet journey, like:

- Almond and coconut flours
- Beef, chicken, or vegetable bouillon cubes
- Canned beans (low sodium)
- Canned diced tomatoes, unsweetened

- Canned light unsweetened coconut milk
- Canned tuna fish or salmon in water
- Ground cinnamon
- Ground pepper
- Salt
- Stevia, finely granulated sweetener, or erythritol
- Whey or pea protein powder

Organize your pantry and shelves. Once you have your staples on hand, organize your kitchen for easy access. When foods and drinks are easy to find, then you're more likely to consume them. Put everything at eye level that you will need for your daily recipes. It will help to have one shelf in your refrigerator for the items you will use frequently, like nonfat, plain, unsweetened Greek yogurt; low-fat milk; eggs; tofu; or low-fat to nonfat cottage cheese. Place meats and seafood on the bottom shelf of your refrigerator to prevent contamination of other foods with any possible drippings.

Pantry Swaps

Use the chart below to replace typical items you may have in your pantry with ones that will be more suitable for your diet after surgery.

BEFORE SURGERY	NOW
Canola oil	Olive oil
Sugar	Stevia or erythritol*
Wheat flour	Almond or coconut flour
Canned fruit in syrup	Canned fruit with no sugar added or in its own juice
Boxed cereal	Oatmeal
Cola	Flavored or plain uncarbonated water
Canned baked beans	Canned low-sodium beans, no seasoning
Tomato sauce	Canned, unsweetened diced tomatoes
Tuna fish in oil	Tuna fish in water
Barbecue sauce	Sugar-free barbecue sauce

CONTINUES »

BEFORE SURGERY	NOW
Mayonnaise	Fat-free or light mayonnaise, unsweetened plain non-fat Greek yogurt, or mashed avocado
Peanut butter	Unsweetened, unsalted peanut butter
Teriyaki sauce	Coconut aminos
Ketchup	Mustard or low-sugar ketchup
Bottled creamy salad dressing	Low-sugar, low-fat vinaigrette salad dressing**

When it comes to sugar alcohols, or those sugars ending in "-tol," you should consume less than 10 grams per serving to prevent digestive symptoms like cramping, abdominal pain, diarrhea, or gas.
**You can also make your own salad dressings with nonfat, plain, unsweetened Greek yogurt and tofu.*

MVP Tools and Equipment

There are certain kitchen tools and equipment that will help you better navigate the post-op diet.

- **Blender:** A high-speed blender will be vital to making smoothies and purees during the first few stages of your post-op diet.
- **Cooking pot with steamer basket:** A pot with a steamer basket makes it easy to steam your vegetables so you don't have to boil them and potentially lose some nutrients in the water.
- **Food processor:** If you have a blender, then a food processor may not be necessary, but it can help in making dressings, sauces, and purees.
- **Vegetable peeler and/or spiralizer:** A vegetable peeler or spiralizer will help you prep vegetables in making soups, purees, and vegetable pasta alternatives during your post-op diet.
- **Vegetable ricer:** Rather than using a whisk, this device will make it easier to rice your steamed cauliflower or broccoli.

HEALTHY EATING HABITS

So far, you've learned a bit about what foods you should eat during your post-op journey. But knowing what to eat is half of the battle; knowing how to eat is the other. That's why it's important to create certain habits around eating that will make long-term success easier.

Meal Planning and Prepping

Meal planning takes some time up-front but can save you time long-term. Take about an hour each week to plan your meals and snacks for the next week. Write down ingredients you'll need that you don't already have on hand. Then use this list as your shopping list. You can wash, peel, and prep veggies and fruit as soon as you return from the grocery store, then store them in sealed containers or freezer bags in the refrigerator until you're ready to cook. Batch-cooking staple items, like cauliflower rice or scrambled eggs, is a great way to have healthy staples on hand to make meals easier and faster.

Mealtime Tips

Take time to sit down and enjoy your meal without distractions. Being distracted, like eating when you're watching television, can cause you to eat faster. It can also cause you to eat larger portions than if you sat and focused on your food.

When you sit down to eat your food, take at least 20 to 30 minutes per meal if you can. Eating too fast can cause digestive distress and may increase the risk of nausea and vomiting. Try chewing your food about 20 to 30 times per bite to slow down your eating and to aid proper digestion. Using a child-size utensil can help you eat smaller bites, which can also support healthy digestion.

Tackling Emotional Eating

Having bariatric surgery is an exciting time but can also be a stressful time for some. This is because eating habits you've had your whole life suddenly change. This can cause stress and lead to emotional eating, which in turn can cause real health consequences, so it's important to learn to manage it.

If you're stressed, call a friend and family member so you can talk your stress out. Or contact a trusted counselor or someone from your healthcare team to receive coping mechanisms. Relaxation breathing, meditation, or yoga can also help manage stress, so you can calm down instead of reaching for food.

Tracking Results

Tracking your results is vital to your success, especially in the early stages. Keeping a food diary in a small notebook or on your smartphone in a food journal app can help you ensure you're eating enough nutrients each day, drinking enough water, and taking your vitamins. You can also track your blood sugar, blood pressure, and weight if you choose. Tracking can remind you now and then how far you've come.

Lifestyle Changes

Making so many changes during your bariatric surgery journey can be overwhelming. But remember that eating isn't the whole journey. Equally important is being healthy in all aspects of your life. Below are tips to create the healthiest lifestyle possible.

Find a support group. Your surgery center may already have a support group where you can meet other people who have had bariatric surgery. These meetings give you the chance to voice concerns and questions with others, as well as with members of your surgical team. You can also access bariatric surgery blogs online for support, but please save any symptom-related questions or concerns for your surgical team.

Move consistently. Staying active is an important part of any lifestyle. It may be difficult to exercise much in the early weeks and months post-op due to your body healing. However, moving in any way a little each day can keep your heart strong and put you on a path to regular exercise. Over time, this can help you meet your long-term health goals. Meeting with a physical therapist can help you find exercises safe for you to do while healing.

Get your Zs. Sleeping at least seven hours each night for most adults is just as important to your health as healthy eating and exercise. Research shows that people who don't sleep enough each night are more likely to gain weight than those who sleep enough. This is likely due to a change in hormone levels when you sleep that is not achieved when you lose sleep. If you have trouble sleeping,

CONTINUES »

ask your doctor to see if a medical issue such as chronic pain, frequent urination during the night, or some other issue may be affecting your sleep.

Practice self-compassion. This post-op journey is not an easy one, so be kind to yourself on both your good days and bad days. One bad day or week doesn't mean that you won't be successful in the long term. Just brush yourself off and put yourself back on track. And don't hesitate to ask for help and support from others if you need it.

ABOUT THE RECIPES

Now that you've learned the basics of what to eat and how to manage your post-op journey, it's time for the recipes. From post-op to general diet, the following pages are full of delicious recipes that will help you consume the protein you need while also enjoying success on your post-op bariatric diet. These recipes will also include:

Familiar favorites: All the recipes are optimized for post-surgery nutrition, but they'll also remind you of some of your favorite foods, such as pizza, chowders, tacos, and pasta dishes, but in a healthy form safe to eat on your post-op diet.

Yields: Servings of most entrées and broths are for four or more, so you can have enough to provide you healthy meals for several days or enough to share meals with loved ones. Smoothies, purees, and snacks are mostly in 1 to 2 servings per recipe.

Serving recommendations: Portion sizes will be specified per every applicable stage. This will save you from having to wonder what an appropriate and safe portion size will be, no matter what stage of the diet you're currently on.

Nutritional information: Every recipe will include nutritional information, so you know what you're getting per serving.

Tips: Each recipe will include tips for cooking, storage, and/or serving. Some recipes will even provide advice on how you can modify the recipe to make it a preferred flavor or to reduce sodium or carbohydrates.

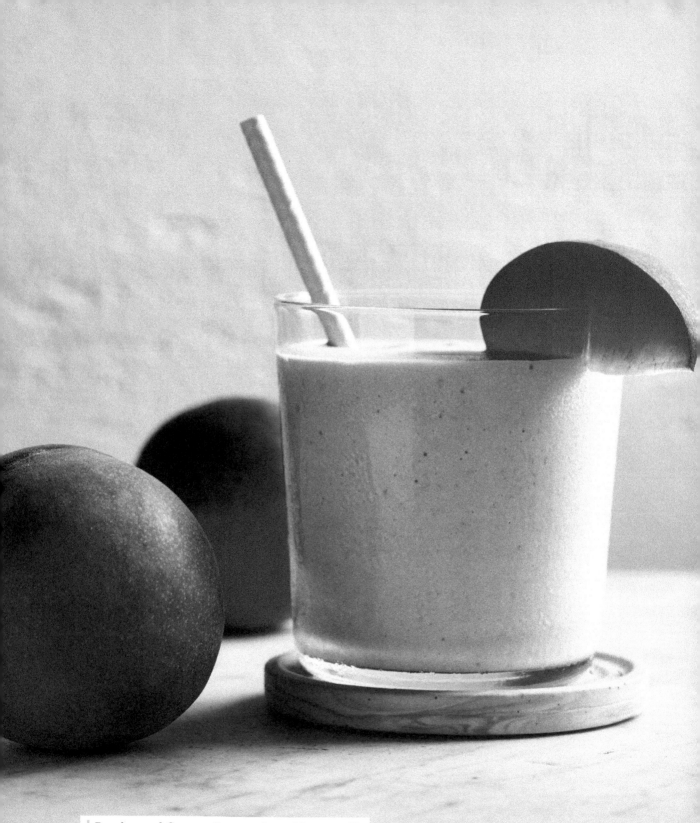

Peaches and Creamy Coconut Smoothie, page 28

Early Post-Op Foods

Savory Beef Bone Broth

MAKES 8 CUPS / PREP TIME: 5 MINUTES / COOK TIME: 5 TO 8 HOURS

When you're post-op and can't enjoy solid foods like a juicy steak, this beef bone broth will help satisfy your cravings safely. Infused with roasted beef and vegetables, this slow-simmered bone broth provides a sippable and flavorful source of protein that's a lower-sodium broth option.

Nonstick cooking spray

1 medium yellow
  onion, chopped

1 cup diced celery

1 cup peeled, diced carrot

3 pounds beef bones

1 pound stew beef

12 cups water

1 teaspoon salt

2 bay leaves

1 tablespoon minced garlic

Serving Recommendations

LIQUID: 2 tablespoons
to ¼ cup

PUREE: ¼ to ½ cup

SOFT FOODS: ½ cup to 1 cup

GENERAL: As tolerated

1. Preheat the oven to 400°F. Coat a shallow roasting pan with cooking spray and set aside.

2. Arrange the onion, celery, and carrot in an even layer in the roasting pan. Place the beef bones and stew beef in the pan on top of the vegetables. Roast the bones, meat, and vegetables for 40 minutes, flipping the meat and bones halfway through the cooking time.

3. Remove the pan from the oven and place the bones, meat, and vegetables into a large stock pot. Add the water, salt, bay leaves, and garlic and bring to a rolling boil.

4. Reduce the heat to medium low and simmer for at least 4 hours. Supervise the pot during the simmering process, stirring a few times an hour.

5. Using a strainer spoon, remove the bones, meat, and vegetables from the pot. Enjoy the broth warm.

STORAGE TIP: Store the leftover bone broth in an airtight container in the refrigerator for up to 3 days or freeze for up to 1 year.

PER SERVING (2 CUPS BROTH): Calories: 138; Protein: 13g; Fat: 8g; Carbohydrates: 2g; Fiber: <1g; Sugar: 0g; Sodium: 465mg

Harvest Vegetable Chicken Bone Broth

MAKES 8 CUPS / PREP TIME: 5 MINUTES / COOK TIME: 5 TO 8 HOURS

If you're craving a hot bowl of chicken soup, this bone broth is the answer without any worry of having to digest solid foods. A simple simmer of roasted carrots, onions, chicken bones, and seasonings such as bay leaves and salt produces a savory flavor that's sure to please your palate and provide plenty of protein.

Nonstick cooking spray

2 cups diced celery

1 medium yellow
   onion, sliced

4 large carrots, peeled
   and chopped

1 (5- to 7-pound)
   whole chicken

12 to 16 cups water

1 teaspoon salt

2 bay leaves

Serving Recommendations

LIQUID: 2 tablespoons
to ¼ cup

PUREE: ¼ to ½ cup

SOFT FOODS: ½ cup to 1 cup

GENERAL: As tolerated

1. Preheat the oven to 400°F. Coat a shallow roasting pan with cooking spray.

2. Arrange the celery, onion, and carrot in the roasting pan. Place the whole raw chicken in the pan. Roast for 90 minutes or more (about 20 minutes per pound of chicken), until a thermometer inserted in the thigh reads 165°F and the juices run clear.

3. Remove the pan from the oven and remove the meat from carcass, setting aside for other recipes.

4. Place the carcass and vegetables in a large pot. Add enough water to the pot to cover the carcass and vegetables completely. Add the salt and bay leaves to the pot and bring to a rolling boil.

5. Simmer over medium heat for at least 4 hours, or longer for increased flavor. Supervise the pot during the simmering process, stirring a few times an hour.

6. Use a strainer spoon to remove the bones and vegetables from the pot. Enjoy the broth warm.

STORAGE TIP: Store the leftover bone broth in an airtight container for up to 3 days or freeze for up to 1 year. You can use the chicken and veggies for another meal option, such as Harvest Vegetable Chicken Soup (page 104); store separately in an airtight container for up to 3 days.

PER SERVING (2 CUPS BROTH): Calories: 138; Protein: 15g; Fat: 2g; Carbohydrates: <1g; Fiber: 0g; Sugar: 0g; Sodium: 400mg

Southwest-Style Chicken Bone Broth

MAKES 8 CUPS / PREP TIME: 5 MINUTES / COOK TIME: 5 TO 8 HOURS

A piping hot bowl of chili is a classic comfort food any time of year. If you're still on a liquid diet, this chili-inspired bone broth will satisfy your craving. Create the taste of your favorite chili or Southwestern-style meal with a simple simmer of low-carbohydrate vegetables, chicken, and seasonings such as bay leaf, cilantro, cumin, and salt.

Nonstick cooking spray
4 large carrots, peeled and chopped
1 medium red onion, quartered
1 large tomato, quartered
1 red bell pepper, sliced
1 (5- to 7-pound) whole chicken
12 to 16 cups water
1 teaspoon salt
1 teaspoon ground cumin
1 teaspoon dried cilantro
2 bay leaves

Serving Recommendations
LIQUID: 2 tablespoons to ¼ cup

PUREE: ¼ to ½ cup

SOFT FOODS: ½ cup to 1 cup

GENERAL: As tolerated

1. Preheat the oven to 400°F. Coat a shallow broiler pan with nonstick cooking spray.

2. Arrange the carrot, onion, tomato, and bell pepper in an even layer in the pan. Place the chicken in the pan and roast for 90 minutes or more (about 20 minutes per pound of chicken), until a thermometer inserted in the thigh reads 165°F and the juices run clear.

3. Remove the pan from the oven and remove the meat from carcass, setting aside for other recipes.

4. Place the carcass and vegetables in a large pot. Add enough water to the pot to cover the carcass and vegetables completely. Add the salt, cumin, cilantro, and bay leaves to the pot and bring to a rolling boil.

5. Reduce the heat to medium and simmer for at least 4 hours, or longer for increased flavor. Supervise the pot during the simmering process, stirring a few times an hour.

6. Use a strainer spoon to remove the bones, meat, and vegetables from the pot. Enjoy the broth warm.

STORAGE TIP: Store the leftover bone broth in an airtight container for up to 3 days or freeze for up to 1 year.

PER SERVING (2 CUPS BROTH): Calories: 138; Protein: 15g; Fat: 2g; Carbohydrates: <1g; Fiber: 0g; Sugar: 0g; Sodium: 400mg

Blueberry Vanilla Smoothie

SERVES 1 / PREP TIME: 5 MINUTES

Enjoy the refreshing taste of blueberries without the common carb-laden breakfast muffin. And as an added bonus, this smoothie gives you the protein-rich content of Greek yogurt and whey protein.

¾ cup nonfat plain Greek yogurt

½ cup fresh or frozen blueberries

1 tablespoon unsweetened vanilla whey protein powder

¼ teaspoon stevia *(optional)*

1. Add the yogurt, blueberries, protein powder, and stevia (if using) to a blender.

2. Blend on low for about 2 minutes until completely combined. Enjoy immediately.

PER SERVING (1 CUP): Calories: 185; Protein: 29g; Fat: 0g; Carbohydrates: 18g; Fiber: 3g; Sugar: 13g; Sodium: 95mg

Serving Recommendations

LIQUID: 2 tablespoons to ¼ cup

PUREE: ¼ to ½ cup

SOFT FOODS: ½ cup to 1 cup

GENERAL: As tolerated

Peaches and Creamy Coconut Smoothie

SERVES 2 / PREP TIME: 5 MINUTES

Peaches and cream can be a delicious dessert, but one high in fat and carbohydrates. However, you can enjoy the tart and creamy flavor of peaches and cream with this low-carbohydrate, high-protein smoothie. Feel free to use any vanilla protein powder you prefer, but I recommend my favorite brand, Integrated Supplements CFM Whey Protein Isolate Powder in vanilla flavor. If you prefer a vegan protein powder, I recommend Orgain Organic Protein plant-based powder in vanilla bean flavor.

¾ cup nonfat plain
  Greek yogurt
¾ cup frozen peaches
¼ cup coconut cream
2 tablespoons
  unsweetened vanilla
  whey protein powder
¼ teaspoon stevia
  (optional)

1. Add the yogurt, peaches, coconut cream, protein powder, and stevia (if using) to a blender.

2. Blend on low for about 2 minutes until completely combined. Enjoy immediately.

STORAGE TIP: If you aren't going to consume immediately, store in the refrigerator in a tightly sealed jar or container for 2 to 3 days. Mix well with a spoon before consuming in case ingredients separate during storage.

Serving Recommendations
LIQUID: 2 tablespoons
to ¼ cup

PUREE: ¼ to ½ cup

SOFT FOODS: ½ cup to 1 cup

GENERAL: As tolerated

PER SERVING (1 CUP): Calories: 162; Protein: 19g; Fat: 4g; Carbohydrates: 13g; Fiber: 2g; Sugar: 10g; Sodium: 67mg

Peanut Butter and Banana Power Smoothie

SERVES 2 / PREP TIME: 5 MINUTES

This smoothie is so protein packed that just one serving provides over 20 grams of protein. The protein in the whey protein powder and peanut butter balances out the carbohydrates from the banana to help support healthy blood glucose balance. If the banana is too much sugar for your tolerance, you can remove it from the recipe for about 90 calories and 12 grams less sugar per serving. For the peanut butter powder, I recommend PB & Me sugar-free peanut butter powder.

1 cup nonfat plain
  Greek yogurt
1 small banana
½ cup ice
¼ cup unsweetened dry
  peanut butter powder
1 tablespoon unsweetened
  vanilla whey
  protein powder
¼ teaspoon stevia
  (optional)

Serving Recommendations
LIQUID: 2 tablespoons
to ¼ cup
PUREE: ¼ to ½ cup
SOFT FOODS: ½ cup to 1 cup
GENERAL: As tolerated

1. Add the yogurt, banana, ice, peanut butter powder, protein powder, and stevia (if using) to a blender.

2. Blend on low for about 2 minutes until completely combined. Enjoy immediately.

> **STORAGE TIP:** Store in an airtight container for up to 2 days in the refrigerator and stir before serving.

PER SERVING (1 CUP): Calories: 178; Protein: 24g; Fat: 2g; Carbohydrates: 20g; Fiber: 4g; Sugar: 12g; Sodium: 88mg

Lemon Meringue Pie Smoothie

SERVES 1 / PREP TIME: 5 MINUTES

Enjoy the sweet and decadent taste of lemon meringue pie in a high-protein, low-carbohydrate smoothie. This creamy, sweet, and tart smoothie is a perfect healthy alternative when your sweet tooth craves dessert.

¾ cup nonfat plain
  Greek yogurt

½ cup unsweetened
  almond milk

Juice of 1 large lemon or
  2 small lemons

1 tablespoon unsweetened
  vanilla whey
  protein powder

1 teaspoon vanilla extract

¼ teaspoon stevia

Serving Recommendations

LIQUID: 2 tablespoons
to ¼ cup

PUREE: ¼ to ½ cup

SOFT FOODS: ½ cup to 1 cup

GENERAL: As tolerated

1. Add the yogurt, almond milk, lemon juice, protein powder, vanilla extract, and stevia to a blender.

2. Blend on low for about 1 minute until completely combined. Enjoy immediately.

> **COOKING TIP:** If you have problems with protein clumping in your smoothie, mix the whey protein powder with almond milk by hand with a fork or whisk first. Then combine this protein shake mixture with yogurt and stevia well, using the same fork or whisk, before adding to the blender.

PER SERVING (1 CUP): Calories: 179; Protein: 29g; Fat: 1g; Carbohydrates: 14g; Fiber: 1g; Sugar: 8g; Sodium: 185mg

Refreshing Strawberry Smoothie

SERVES 1 / PREP TIME: 5 MINUTES

If you need some fruit-flavored refreshment but are trying to avoid high-sugar juice drinks, this smoothie will fit the bill. Blended with nonfat Greek yogurt, this refreshing smoothie also provides a rich source of protein to help you stay full until your next meal.

1 cup nonfat plain
   Greek yogurt
1 cup frozen unsweetened
   strawberries
¼ teaspoon stevia

Serving Recommendations
LIQUID: 2 tablespoons
to ¼ cup

PUREE: ¼ to ½ cup

SOFT FOODS: ½ cup to 1 cup

GENERAL: As tolerated

1. Add the yogurt, strawberries, and stevia to a blender.

2. Blend on low for about 2 minutes until completely combined. Enjoy immediately.

COOKING TIP: If you prefer a thinner smoothie, add a few tablespoons of unsweetened almond milk before blending.

PER SERVING (2 CUPS): Calories: 170; Protein: 24g; Fat: 0g; Carbohydrates: 20g; Fiber: 3g; Sugar: 16g; Sodium: 87mg

Creamy Pumpkin Pie Smoothie

SERVES 1 / PREP TIME: 5 MINUTES

Pumpkin spice is a fall classic that you don't have to wait until fall to enjoy. The sweet cinnamon flavor of this pumpkin pie smoothie balanced with vanilla whey protein and creamy Greek yogurt makes for a delicious meal option any time of day.

1 cup nonfat plain
  Greek yogurt
⅔ cup unsweetened
  canned pumpkin
1 tablespoon unsweetened
  vanilla whey
  protein powder
1¼ teaspoon ground
  cinnamon
½ teaspoon stevia
  (optional)
Dash salt (optional)

1. Add the yogurt, pumpkin, protein powder, cinnamon, stevia (if using), and salt (if using) to a blender.

2. Blend on low for about 2 minutes until completely combined. Enjoy immediately.

> **COOKING TIP:** If you prefer a spicier pumpkin pie flavor, add more cinnamon and/or a bit of nutmeg.

PER SERVING (1½ CUPS): Calories: 242; Protein: 36g; Fat: 1g; Carbohydrates: 25g; Fiber: 7g; Sugar: 14g; Sodium: 180mg

Serving Recommendations
LIQUID: 2 tablespoons
to ¼ cup

PUREE: ¼ to ½ cup

SOFT FOODS: ½ cup to 1 cup

GENERAL: As tolerated

Neapolitan Smoothie

SERVES 1 / PREP TIME: 5 MINUTES

This Neapolitan ice cream–inspired smoothie is reminiscent of melted Neapolitan flavored ice cream, hence its name. This blend of strawberries, cocoa, and vanilla flavors mixed with creamy Greek yogurt provide a uniquely sweet taste in a protein-rich and low-carbohydrate form.

1 cup nonfat plain
   Greek yogurt
½ cup fresh or frozen
   strawberries
¼ cup unsweetened
   almond milk
½ tablespoon unsweetened
   cocoa powder
1 teaspoon vanilla extract
¼ teaspoon stevia
   (optional)

Serving Recommendations
LIQUID: 2 tablespoons
to ¼ cup

PUREE: ¼ to ½ cup

SOFT FOODS: ½ cup to 1 cup

GENERAL: As tolerated

1. Add the yogurt, strawberries, almond milk, cocoa powder, vanilla extract, and stevia (if using) to a blender.

2. Blend on low for about 2 minutes until completely combined. Enjoy immediately.

> **COOKING TIP:** Feel free to add 1 tablespoon of vanilla-, chocolate-, or strawberry-flavored unsweetened protein powder for extra protein content.

PER SERVING (1½ CUPS): Calories: 189; Protein: 24g; Fat: 2g; Carbohydrates: 20g; Fiber: 5g; Sugar: 12g; Sodium: 115mg

Cinnamon Apple Pie Smoothie

SERVES 1 / PREP TIME: 5 MINUTES

This creamy, delicious smoothie was inspired by the holiday favorite of hot apple pie. The best part is that, unlike its muse, this smoothie is low in sugar and high in protein and flavor. And you don't even have to preheat the oven to enjoy this dessert-like beverage.

1 cup peeled and
   sliced apple
⅔ cup nonfat plain
   Greek yogurt
1 tablespoon unsweetened
   vanilla whey
   protein powder
1 teaspoon ground
   cinnamon
¼ teaspoon stevia
   (optional)

Serving Recommendations
LIQUID: 2 tablespoons
to ¼ cup

PUREE: ¼ to ½ cup

SOFT FOODS: ½ cup to 1 cup

GENERAL: As tolerated

1. Add the apple, yogurt, protein powder, cinnamon, and stevia (if using) to a blender.

2. Blend on high for about 2 minutes or until thoroughly combined. Enjoy immediately.

> **INGREDIENT TIP:** The type of apple you use will depend on your preference for tart or sweet. Fuji or Gala apples will be sweet, Honey Crisp or Pink Lady apples will be sweet-tart, and Granny Smith apples will be very tart.

PER SERVING (1¼ CUP): Calories: 183; Protein: 26g; Fat: 1g; Carbohydrates: 20g; Fiber: 3g; Sugar: 14g; Sodium: 143mg

Tuna-Avocado Salad

SERVES 1 / PREP TIME: 5 MINUTES

Enjoy tuna fish without the excess fat from mayonnaise. Using avocado instead of mayonnaise adds fiber and healthy fats that help enhance the health of your body while providing a tasty lunch or dinner meal option. Feel free to remove onion from the recipe if you prefer or if the texture is not tolerated well.

6 tablespoons canned
  tuna, drained

2 tablespoons
  mashed avocado

2 tablespoons diced
  red onion

Squeeze of lemon juice

⅛ teaspoon dried cilantro

Salt *(optional)*

Freshly ground black
  pepper *(optional)*

Serving Recommendations
PUREE: ¼ to ½ cup (blend mixture until smooth before serving)

SOFT FOODS: ½ cup to 1 cup

GENERAL: As tolerated

1. Add the tuna, avocado, onion, lemon juice, and cilantro to a blender. Season with salt (if using) and pepper (if using) to taste.

2. Blend on low for about 1 minute or until completely combined. Enjoy immediately.

3. Store the leftover salad in an airtight container in the refrigerator for up to 3 days.

PER SERVING (½ CUP): Calories: 113; Protein: 17g; Fat: 4g; Carbohydrates: 5g; Fiber: 2g; Sugar: 1g; Sodium: 212mg

Roasted Carrot Puree

SERVES 4 / PREP TIME: 5 MINUTES / COOK TIME: 30 MINUTES

Creamy soups can be comforting but are high in fat that your body may not tolerate. But that doesn't mean you can't enjoy a creamy meal. This puree gives you a thick and creamy consistency and the satisfying flavor of carrot without all the fat, but with plenty of protein.

1 cup peeled, sliced carrot

½ tablespoon extra-virgin olive oil

Dash salt

¾ cup nonfat plain Greek yogurt

¼ cup unsweetened almond milk

Serving Recommendations

PUREE: ¼ to ½ cup

SOFT FOODS: ½ cup to 1 cup

GENERAL: As tolerated

1. Preheat the oven to 425°F. Line a baking sheet with parchment paper and set aside.

2. In a bowl, toss the carrot and oil. Arrange the carrot slices on the prepared baking sheet and sprinkle with salt.

3. Bake for 25 to 30 minutes, until the carrot softens and starts to turn golden brown.

4. Add the carrot, yogurt, and almond milk to a blender. Blend on low for about a minute or so, until the mixture turns bright orange. Enjoy.

5. Store the leftover puree in an airtight container in the refrigerator for up to 5 days.

SERVING TIP: Warm in the microwave for about 30 to 60 seconds after blending and before serving, since the addition of yogurt will cool down the cooked carrots.

PER SERVING (3½ TABLESPOONS): Calories: 44; Protein: 4g; Fat: 2g; Carbohydrates: 3g; Fiber: 1g; Sugar: 2g; Sodium: 75mg

Broccoli-Cheddar Puree

SERVES 4 / PREP TIME: 5 MINUTES / COOK TIME: 5 MINUTES

Broccoli and cheese can be a delicious side dish, but if you're not able to eat fibrous foods just yet, they are off-limits—until now. Blend together some protein-rich cottage cheese, shredded cheddar, and steamed broccoli to get an easy-to-digest form of this comfort food favorite.

2 cups diced
   broccoli florets
⅔ cup low-fat
   cottage cheese
⅓ cup part-skim shredded
   Cheddar cheese

Serving Recommendations

PUREE: ¼ to ½ cup

SOFT FOODS: ½ cup to 1 cup

GENERAL: As tolerated

1. Fill the bottom of a medium saucepan with a couple inches of water and insert a steamer basket. Place the broccoli in the steamer basket and bring the water to a boil. Cover and steam for 5 minutes or until tender. Remove from the heat.

2. Add the broccoli, cottage cheese, and Cheddar cheese to a blender or food processor. Blend the mixture for about 2 minutes or until smooth. Enjoy.

3. Store the leftover puree in an airtight container in the refrigerator for up to 5 days.

COOKING TIP: If you prefer, you can use broccoli that you can steam in a bag if you wish to save some prep time. Just make sure there are no sauce or seasonings added. Also, for a different flavor, replace the broccoli with cauliflower or use a different cheese like Parmesan instead of Cheddar.

PER SERVING (¾ CUP): Calories: 78; Protein: 8g; Fat: 3g; Carbohydrates: 7g; Fiber: 2g; Sugar: 3g; Sodium: 175mg

Butternut Squash Puree

SERVES 4 / PREP TIME: 5 MINUTES / COOK TIME: 15 MINUTES

This fall favorite vegetable blends deliciously well with Greek yogurt and cheese to give you a creamy soup sure to please your palate. And the addition of a few spices like sage, garlic powder, and salt give it just enough subtle flavor to make it taste like your favorite autumn soup.

2 cups diced
   butternut squash
1 cup nonfat plain
   Greek yogurt
½ cup shredded
   Parmesan cheese
½ teaspoon garlic powder
¼ teaspoon dried sage
¼ teaspoon salt

Serving Recommendations
PUREE: ¼ to ½ cup
SOFT FOODS: ½ cup to 1 cup
GENERAL: As tolerated

1. Fill the bottom of a medium saucepan with a couple inches of water and insert a steamer basket. Place the squash in the steamer basket and bring the water to a boil. Cover and steam for 15 minutes or until soft. Remove from the heat.

2. Add the butternut squash, yogurt, Parmesan cheese, garlic powder, sage, and salt to a blender or food processor. Blend the mixture for about 2 minutes or until smooth. Enjoy.

3. Store the leftover puree in an airtight container in the refrigerator for up to 5 days.

> **COOKING TIP:** If you prefer, you can use butternut squash that you can steam in a bag if you wish to save some prep time. Just make sure there are no sauce or seasonings added.

PER SERVING (¾ CUP): Calories: 104; Protein: 11g; Fat: 3g; Carbohydrates: 11g; Fiber: 2g; Sugar: 3g; Sodium: 339mg

Cheese Pizza Puree

SERVES 4 / PREP TIME: 5 MINUTES / COOK TIME: 5 MINUTES

Cheesy pizza is a favorite food of many, especially on weekends and special nights out. But unfortunately, it can be dripping with fat, while the crust brings more carbohydrates to the table than you should be eating in your healthy diet. This cheese pizza puree recipe takes the toppings off that crust, lowers the fat, and blends it into an easy-to-digest form. If you prefer, add in garlic powder and/or Italian seasoning for extra flavor.

½ cup unsweetened almond milk

1 tablespoon cornstarch

1 cup part-skim shredded mozzarella cheese

1 cup canned diced tomatoes, drained

Dash salt

Serving Recommendations

PUREE: 4 to 8 tablespoons

SOFT FOODS: 8 to 16 tablespoons (1 to 2 full servings)

GENERAL: As tolerated

1. In a medium saucepan, heat the almond milk over medium heat. Whisk in the cornstarch and bring the mixture to a rolling boil.

2. Reduce the heat to low-medium and mix in the mozzarella cheese a few tablespoons at a time, stirring continuously.

3. Once the cheese is melted and combined with the milk, remove the pan from the heat and set aside to cool slightly.

4. Place the tomato and salt in a blender and blend on low for about 30 seconds or until smooth.

5. In a large serving bowl, combine the cheese and tomato mixtures and enjoy.

> **STORAGE TIP:** Store leftovers in an airtight container in the refrigerator for 3 to 4 days.

PER SERVING (7 TABLESPOONS): Calories: 104; Protein: 8g; Fat: 6g; Carbohydrates: 6g; Fiber: 1g; Sugar: 2g; Sodium: 321mg

Potato and Cheddar Mash Puree

SERVES 5 / PREP TIME: 5 MINUTES / COOK TIME: 15 MINUTES

Mashed potatoes are a comfort classic but can be high in calories, carbohydrates, and fat due to their usual milk- and butter-laden content. However, it doesn't have to be this way. Enjoy the creamy goodness of mashed potatoes with cheese in a protein-rich form that can satisfy your mashed potato cravings. To save time on prep, you can use frozen cubed potatoes (no sauce or seasoning added) in place of fresh.

2 cups peeled, diced russet potatoes (2½ medium potatoes)

1 cup part-skim shredded Cheddar cheese

1 cup nonfat plain Greek yogurt

Serving Recommendations

PUREE: 4 to 8 tablespoons

SOFT FOODS: 8 to 16 tablespoons (1 to 2 full servings)

GENERAL: As tolerated

1. Fill the bottom of a medium saucepan with a couple inches of water and insert a steamer basket. Place the potatoes in the steamer basket, bring the water to a boil, cover, and steam for about 15 minutes, until softened. Remove from the heat.

2. Add the potatoes, Cheddar cheese, and yogurt to a blender or food processor. Blend the mixture on low for about 2 minutes or until smooth. Enjoy.

STORAGE TIP: Store leftovers in an airtight container in the refrigerator for 3 to 4 days.

PER SERVING (½ CUP): Calories: 144; Protein: 11g; Fat: 7g; Carbohydrates: 10g; Fiber: 1g; Sugar: 1g; Sodium: 300mg

Harvest Vegetable Chicken Puree

SERVES 4 / PREP TIME: 5 MINUTES / COOK TIME: 25 MINUTES

If you wish you could have a bowl of chicken noodle soup, but pasta or solid foods are off-limits, this recipe takes aspects of the Harvest Vegetable Chicken Soup (page 104) and blends it to a perfectly easy-to-digest texture without sacrificing flavor. To cook the chicken, bring a few cups of water to a boil and simmer a half-pound chicken breast for about 25 minutes, until cooked through, then shred with two forks.

1 tablespoon extra-virgin olive oil

2 cups peeled, thinly sliced carrot

½ cup diced yellow onion

1 cup shredded chicken breast

1 cup chicken broth, store-bought or Harvest Vegetable Chicken Bone Broth (page 25)

¼ teaspoon salt

Serving Recommendations
PUREE: 4 to 8 tablespoons

SOFT FOODS: 8 to 16 tablespoons (1 to 2 full servings)

GENERAL: As tolerated

1. In a large saucepan, heat the oil over medium-high heat. Add the carrot and onion to the pan and cook, stirring every 30 seconds or so, for 7 to 9 minutes, or until the onion is translucent and the carrot is soft. Add a few tablespoons of water if needed to help steam carrot.

2. Add the chicken, broth, and salt to the pan. Simmer for another 7 to 9 minutes on low heat to allow the flavors to develop.

3. Turn off the heat and remove the pan from burner. Allow mixture to cool for 5 to 7 minutes.

4. Place the cooled mixture in a blender or food processor. Blend on low for about 2 minutes or until smooth. Enjoy.

STORAGE TIP: Store leftovers in an airtight container in the refrigerator for 5 to 7 days.

PER SERVING (½ CUP): Calories: 171; Protein: 19g; Fat: 6g; Carbohydrates: 6g; Fiber: 1g; Sugar: 3g; Sodium: 247mg

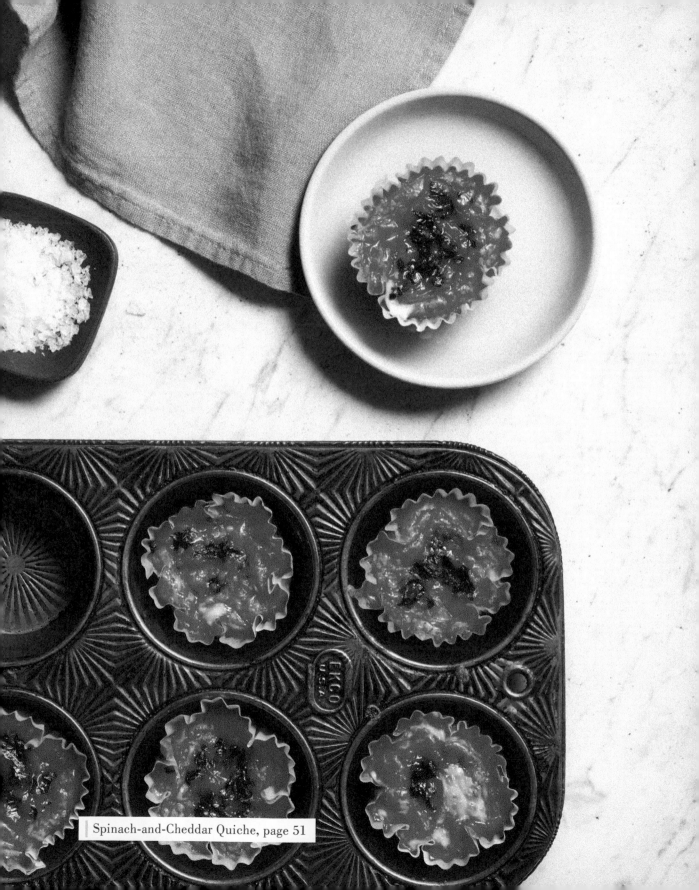

Spinach-and-Cheddar Quiche, page 51

Breakfast Foods

Egg White "Pizza"

SERVES 4 / PREP TIME: 5 MINUTES / COOK TIME: 5 MINUTES

Pizza is high in carbohydrates and fat, which can sabotage your healthy eating efforts and may be hard for post-op bariatric patients to digest. This egg white "pizza" provides all the flavors of your favorite pizza toppings in a protein-rich, low-fat, and low-carbohydrate recipe.

1 tablespoon extra-virgin olive oil

12 large egg whites (1½ cups egg whites)

½ teaspoon Italian seasoning

½ teaspoon garlic powder

¼ teaspoon salt

Nonstick cooking spray (optional)

½ cup shredded mozzarella cheese

1 cup sliced tomato (1 large tomato)

Serving Recommendations

SOFT FOODS: about ¾ cup of food

GENERAL: ¾ to 1½ cups food, depending on your tolerance and calorie needs daily

1. In a large skillet, heat the oil over medium heat.

2. In a large bowl, beat the egg whites with the Italian seasoning, garlic powder, and salt.

3. Pour the mixture into the skillet and cover with a lid. Cook for 1 to 2 minutes, or until egg whites start to bubble. Use a spatula to carefully lift at the edges to ensure the egg whites are not sticking to the skillet. If they are sticking, lower the heat, lift the egg whites from the skillet carefully, and spray with cooking spray before placing the egg whites back in skillet.

4. Remove the lid and sprinkle the mozzarella cheese over the eggs. Place the tomato slices on top. Cover and heat for another 1 or 2 minutes until the cheese melts.

5. Carefully remove the egg white pizza from the pan. Divide into quarters and serve hot.

STORAGE TIP: Store leftovers in an airtight container in the refrigerator for up to 3 days.

PER SERVING (¾ CUP): Calories: 180; Protein: 19g; Fat: 11g; Carbohydrates: 6g; Fiber: 1g; Sugar: 3g; Sodium: 486mg

Southwest Scramble

SERVES 4 / PREP TIME: 5 MINUTES / COOK TIME: 10 MINUTES

If you want to spice up your breakfast, this egg scramble option is the right fit for you. It's like a breakfast burrito without the high-carbohydrate flour tortilla. Top with light sour cream or your favorite salsa for the ultimate Southwest-style breakfast dish. The texture of this dish is good for those on either a soft diet or general diet.

8 teaspoons extra-virgin olive oil

8 large eggs

½ cup diced red or yellow onion

½ cup diced bell pepper

½ cup canned diced tomatoes, drained

¼ teaspoon salt

Dash ground black pepper (optional)

½ cup sliced avocado

Serving Recommendations

PUREE: ¼ to ½ cup

SOFT FOODS: ½ cup to 1 cup (about 1 serving)

GENERAL: 1 to 2 cups (equal to about 2 servings)

1. In a large skillet, heat the oil over medium-high heat.

2. In a medium bowl, beat the eggs well for about 1 minute. Set aside.

3. Add the onion and pepper to the skillet and cook, stirring frequently, for about 5 minutes, until the onion is translucent.

4. Add in the beaten egg and cook for 1 to 2 minutes until the egg is cooked well, stirring frequently.

5. Add in diced tomato and cook for an additional 1 to 2 minutes. Remove from the heat.

6. Sprinkle the scramble with salt and pepper (if using). Top the egg scramble with sliced avocado.

STORAGE TIP: To keep leftover avocado fresh, store in a storage bag in the refrigerator for up to 3 days. After that point, the avocado may start to brown, so try to use it before then to prevent waste. Store leftover eggs in an airtight container in the refrigerator for up to 3 days.

PER SERVING (¾ TO 1 CUP): Calories: 266; Protein: 14g; Fat: 21g; Carbohydrates: 6g; Fiber: 2g; Sugar: 2g; Sodium: 292mg

Italian-Style Scramble

SERVES 4 / PREP TIME: 5 MINUTES / COOK TIME: 5 MINUTES

If you're tired of eating the same old plain eggs for breakfast in the morning, spice it up with some Italian flavor. By adding fresh tomatoes and spices as well as rich and creamy mozzarella, you can turn your basic breakfast into a meal you look forward to each morning.

Nonstick cooking spray

8 large eggs

1 cup canned diced
   tomatoes, drained

1 cup shredded
   mozzarella cheese

1 teaspoon Italian
   seasoning

1 teaspoon garlic powder

¼ teaspoon salt

Serving Recommendations

Puree: ¼ to ½ cup

Soft Foods: ½ cup to 1 cup

General: 1 to 2 servings, depending on your tolerance and calorie needs daily

1. Spray a large skillet with nonstick cooking spray and heat over medium heat.

2. In a large bowl, combine the eggs, tomato, mozzarella cheese, Italian seasoning, garlic powder, and salt and beat well until combined.

3. Pour the mixture into the skillet and cook for 3 to 5 minutes, stirring frequently, until the eggs are set.

4. Remove from the heat and serve.

STORAGE TIP: Store leftovers in an airtight container in the refrigerator for up to 3 days.

PER SERVING (1 CUP): Calories: 241; Protein: 21g; Fat: 16g; Carbohydrates: 6g; Fiber: 1g; Sugar: 2g; Sodium: 577mg

Cheeseburger Scramble

SERVES 4 / PREP TIME: 5 MINUTES / COOK TIME: 10 MINUTES

Bring the taste of a juicy cheeseburger to breakfast with this high-protein, low-carbohydrate scramble. It's easy to make and helps keep mealtime flavorful and healthy at the same time. You can even use cooked ground beef from a leftover dinner meal to make this omelet an even more convenient meal option. Feel free to add other vegetables like diced pepper or onion to the recipe as well.

Nonstick cooking spray

8 ounces lean ground beef

4 large eggs

½ cup canned diced
  tomatoes, drained

½ cup shredded
  Cheddar cheese

¼ teaspoon salt

Serving Recommendations

Soft Foods: ½ cup to 1 cup
(about 1 full serving)

General: 1 to 2 servings
(depending on daily calorie needs)

1. Spray a large skillet with cooking spray and cook the ground beef over medium heat for about 3 minutes, stirring frequently, until fully browned.

2. Remove the beef from heat. Drain the fat into a bowl or jar for disposal, spoon the beef into a separate bowl or plate, and set aside.

3. Place the skillet back over medium heat and spray again with cooking spray. Crack the eggs into a small bowl and beat well. Pour the eggs into skillet and cook for 2 to 3 minutes, stirring frequently, until the eggs are set.

4. Reduce the heat to low. Add the tomato, Cheddar cheese, beef, and salt to the skillet and mix well, allowing the mixture to heat 1 to 2 more minutes, or until cheese is melted.

5. Remove from the heat and serve.

STORAGE TIP: Store leftovers in an airtight container in the refrigerator for up to 3 days.

PER SERVING (⅔ CUP): Calories: 218; Protein: 21g; Fat: 13g; Carbohydrates: 2g; Fiber: <1g; Sugar: 1g; Sodium: 386mg

Butternut Squash and Cauliflower Cheesy Hash Browns

SERVES 4 / PREP TIME: 10 MINUTES / COOK TIME: 50 MINUTES

Whether you call them home fries, fried potatoes, or cottage fries, this morning potato dish pairs great with eggs or sausage. However, it can be high in carbohydrates and fat due to its potato content and typically fried cooking method. By replacing potatoes with low-carbohydrate vegetables like cauliflower and butternut squash, and baking them instead of frying, you can produce a healthy hash brown alternative.

1 tablespoon extra-virgin olive oil

1 cup peeled and diced butternut squash

1 cup cauliflower rice

½ cup water

¼ teaspoon salt

2 large eggs

½ cup shredded Cheddar cheese

½ cup almond flour

Serving Recommendations

PUREE: 1 to 1½ hash browns

SOFT FOODS: about 2 to 3 hash browns (if eating them as your whole meal)

GENERAL: 2 to 4 hash browns (depending on your tolerance and daily calorie needs; 2 cakes if you plan on eating them with another food item)

1. Preheat the oven to 400°F.

2. In a large skillet, heat the oil over medium heat. Add the diced butternut squash and cook for 10 to 12 minutes, stirring frequently.

3. Add the riced cauliflower, water, and salt to the skillet. Cook for 8 to 10 minutes and stir frequently until water is absorbed. Remove from the heat and cool for 5 to 7 minutes.

4. Take a large piece of cheesecloth or clean kitchen towel and drape it open over a large mixing bowl. Then scoop the mixture into the center of the cheesecloth and bring all corners of the cloth together. Over top of the bowl, twist the cloth closed around the mixture and squeeze as much liquid out of the vegetable mixture as possible.

5. Remove the cheesecloth and place the drained mixture back into its original bowl. Add in the eggs, Cheddar cheese, and almond flour and combine ingredients well.

6. Line a baking sheet with parchment paper. To form each patty, gather the mixture into 2 heaping table-spoons and space about 1 inch apart. Flatten each mound of mixture into a round patty shape.

7. Bake the hash browns in the oven for about 20 minutes or until golden brown and crispy.

STORAGE TIP: You can store hash browns in an airtight container for up to 5 days in the refrigerator. To reheat, prepare a baking sheet with aluminum foil, spray with cooking spray, and arrange the hash browns on the baking sheet. Bake for about 7 to 10 minutes at 400°F until crispy on the edges.

PER SERVING (2 HASH BROWNS): Calories: 197; Protein: 11g; Fat: 14g; Carbohydrates: 10g; Fiber: 4g; Sugar: 2g; Sodium: 278mg

Turkey, Zucchini, and Tomato Hash

SERVES 4 / PREP TIME: 5 MINUTES / COOK TIME: 15 MINUTES

This hash uses a foundation of ground turkey and low-carbohydrate zucchini to volumize this unique breakfast option. This recipe provides the basics, but feel free to add extra vegetables of your choice to the hash such as butternut squash, peppers, sweet potatoes, or more of the ingredients already present.

1 tablespoon extra-virgin olive oil

8 ounces lean ground turkey

2 cups zucchini cut into ½-inch dice

1 cup canned diced tomatoes, drained

½ cup diced onion

¼ teaspoon salt

Serving Recommendation
Soft Foods: ½ cup to 1 cup (about 1 full serving)

General: 1 to 2 servings (depending on your daily calorie needs)

1. In a large skillet, heat the oil over medium heat. Place the ground turkey in the skillet and cook, stirring frequently, for about 5 minutes, until browned. Remove the turkey and place in a small bowl. Set aside.

2. Place the zucchini, tomato, and onion in the skillet and cook for 7 to 10 minutes, stirring occasionally, or until the onion is translucent and the zucchini is soft. Add the salt and mix well.

3. Remove from the heat. Combine the turkey and vegetables and serve.

> **STORAGE TIP:** Store leftovers of the hash in an airtight container in the refrigerator for up to 3 days.

PER SERVING (¾ CUP): Calories: 110; Protein: 12g; Fat: 4g; Carbohydrates: 6g; Fiber: 1g; Sugar: 4g; Sodium: 277mg

Spinach-and-Cheddar Quiche

SERVES 4 / PREP TIME: 5 MINUTES / COOK TIME: 25 MINUTES

A breakfast on the go doesn't have to be a sugary muffin or coffee drink. Make these savory spinach-and-cheese quiches the night before and grab a couple for the road if you choose. These portable breakfast bites provide a ton of protein as well as some antioxidant-rich leafy greens for inflammation-fighting power. To save time, you can use steam-in-the-bag spinach for this recipe. Just be sure to drain the spinach well after cooking and before adding to the egg mixture.

Nonstick cooking spray
1 cup chopped spinach
4 large eggs
½ cup shredded
    Cheddar cheese
¼ teaspoon salt

Serving Recommendations
SOFT FOODS: 1 to 2 quiches (equal to ½ to 1 cup)

GENERAL: 2 to 4 quiches (depending on tolerance and daily calorie needs)

1. Preheat the oven to 350°F.

2. Line a muffin tin with 8 cupcake liners and spray each liner with nonstick cooking spray.

3. Fill the bottom of a medium saucepan with a couple inches of water and insert a steamer basket. Bring the water to a boil, then place the spinach in the steamer basket and cook for 3 minutes. Remove from the heat and drain well in a colander, pressing with the back of a spoon to remove the liquid.

4. In a medium mixing bowl, combine the spinach, eggs, Cheddar cheese, and salt. Pour the mixture evenly into the lined cups.

5. Bake for 15 to 20 minutes, or until a toothpick inserted in the middle of a quiche comes out clean. Enjoy warm.

> **STORAGE TIP:** Store leftovers in an airtight container in the refrigerator for up to 3 days.

PER SERVING (2 EGG QUICHES): Calories: 128; Protein: 10g; Fat: 9g; Carbohydrates: 1g; Fiber: <1g; Sugar: <1g; Sodium: 312mg

Cheesecake Cottage Cheese

SERVES 2 / PREP TIME: 2 MINUTES, PLUS 30 MINUTES TO CHILL

The creamy taste of cheesecake provides a comfort food indulgence but can also bring with it a lot of sugar and fat. If you still crave that taste, this protein-rich breakfast meal can fill that void. Pair with your favorite low-carbohydrate fruit like strawberries or blueberries for an extra dose of flavor as well as fiber.

1 cup low-fat
  cottage cheese
2 tablespoons whipped
  cream cheese
2 teaspoons brown sugar
1 teaspoon vanilla extract

Serving Recommendations
PUREE: ¼ to ½ cup

SOFT FOODS: ½ cup to 1 cup
(1 to 2 servings)

GENERAL: 1 to 1½ cups
(depending on your tolerance
and daily needs)

1. In a bowl, combine the cottage cheese, cream cheese, brown sugar, and vanilla extract. Mix well.

2. Serve and enjoy alone or with your favorite low-carbohydrate fruit. Best served chilled in the refrigerator for about 30 minutes before eating.

STORAGE TIP: Store the leftovers in an airtight container in the refrigerator for up to 10 days.

PER SERVING (½ CUP): Calories: 128; Protein: 12g; Fat: 4g; Carbohydrates: 11g; Fiber: 0g; Sugar: 8g; Sodium: 369mg

Mixed Berry Shortcake Yogurt Crumble

SERVES 2 / PREP TIME: 5 MINUTES / COOK TIME: 5 MINUTES

Pie for breakfast sounds too good to be true. Or, at the very least a very unhealthy option—until now. This easy-to-make shortcake-style yogurt parfait brings the sweetness of a fruit crumble dessert to a protein-rich breakfast meal option. Consume alone or use as a topping for Cinnamon Flax-and-Almond Breakfast Cakes (page 57) for a sweet morning meal.

2 tablespoons almond flour

½ teaspoon ground cinnamon

¼ teaspoon stevia

½ tablespoon unsalted butter

2 tablespoons frozen or fresh diced strawberries

2 tablespoons frozen or fresh blueberries

1 cup nonfat plain Greek yogurt

1 teaspoon vanilla extract

Serving Recommendations

PUREE: ¼ to ½ cup (about 1 serving)

SOFT FOODS: ½ cup to 1 cup (about 2 servings)

GENERAL: 1 to 2 servings (depending on your tolerance and daily calorie needs)

1. In a small bowl, combine the almond flour, cinnamon, and stevia.

2. In a small skillet, combine the butter and almond flour mixture over medium heat. Cook for 1 to 2 minutes, stirring frequently as the butter melts. Once the moisture from the butter is absorbed and the mixture starts to crisp and clump a bit, remove the mixture from heat. Set the almond flour mixture aside in a separate bowl and carefully wipe out the skillet.

3. Place the strawberries and blueberries in the skillet and cook for 2 to 3 minutes, stirring frequently until softened. Remove from the heat.

4. In a small bowl, mix the yogurt with the vanilla extract. Layer the yogurt, fruit, and almond flour mixture in two serving bowls and enjoy.

STORAGE TIP: Store leftovers in an airtight container in the refrigerator up to 7 days.

PER SERVING (⅓ CUP): Calories: 147; Protein: 14g; Fat: 7g; Carbohydrates: 11g; Fiber: 2g; Sugar: 8g; Sodium: 44mg

Banana Brûlée Yogurt Parfait

SERVES 1 / PREP TIME: 5 MINUTES / COOK TIME: 2 MINUTES

Have you ever craved dessert for breakfast? If you answered yes, then this is one recipe you'll want to hold onto. The tartness and protein-rich content of the yogurt balanced with the sweetness and rich flavor of the cooked bananas provide a satisfying breakfast meal that could also be consumed for evening dessert.

Nonstick cooking spray
¼ cup banana slices
1 teaspoon brown sugar
1 cup nonfat plain
  Greek yogurt
Dash ground cinnamon

Serving Recommendations
Puree: ¼ to ½ cup
Soft Foods: ½ cup to 1 cup
General: 1 full serving
(1¼ cup)

1. Spray a small skillet with cooking spray. Place over medium heat.

2. Place the banana slices in the skillet. Sprinkle the brown sugar over the banana slices. Cook for 1 to 2 minutes, stirring frequently, until heated through. Remove from the heat.

3. Place the yogurt into a bowl and pour the banana mixture over the yogurt. Sprinkle with cinnamon and enjoy immediately.

COOKING TIP: Be sure to have ingredients measured out prior to cooking the banana slices, as this mixture will cook fast and may burn if you're not careful.

PER SERVING (1¼ CUP): Calories: 168; Protein: 24g; Fat: 0g; Carbohydrates: 20g; Fiber: 1g; Sugar: 16g; Sodium: 88mg

Cinnamon-Spice Overnight Cereal

SERVES 1 / PREP TIME: 5 MINUTES, PLUS OVERNIGHT CHILLING

If you're rushing around in the morning and don't have time to make a healthy breakfast, this is a simple, tasty solution. Set aside a few minutes before you go to bed to assemble a jar of overnight oats so that you can wake up, grab it from the refrigerator, and enjoy before you start your day.

¾ cup nonfat plain
   Greek yogurt
4 tablespoons
   unsweetened
   almond milk
3 tablespoons almond flour
2 tablespoons quick oats
1 tablespoon chia seeds
1 teaspoon ground
   cinnamon
¼ teaspoon stevia

Serving Recommendations
Puree: ¼ to ½ cup

Soft Foods: ½ cup to 1 cup

General: 1 full serving (a little over 1 cup)

1. In a pint-size canning jar, combine the yogurt, almond milk, almond flour, oats, chia seeds, cinnamon, and stevia.

2. Seal tightly and place in the refrigerator. Allow the oat mixture to sit overnight for at least 8 hours to set.

3. Enjoy cold or remove the lid and heat in the microwave for about 30 seconds to warm before eating. If consuming only a portion of the recipe, you may need to check smaller portions (½ cup or less) every 10 seconds to prevent overcooking.

STORAGE TIP: A canning jar with a tightly sealed lid works best for this recipe, especially if you plan on taking the cereal mixture with you on the go. This type of jar, with the lid removed, is also microwave safe.

PER SERVING (1 CUP): Calories: 336; Protein: 27g; Fat: 17g; Carbohydrates: 26g; Fiber: 9g; Sugar: 6g; Sodium: 111mg

PB and J Overnight No-Oats Cereal

SERVES 2 / PREP TIME: 5 MINUTES, PLUS OVERNIGHT CHILLING /
COOK TIME: 2 MINUTES

If you love peanut butter and jelly but want to cut down on carbohydrates, enjoy these traditional flavors in your morning cereal. And if you're not sure you have time in the morning to prepare this delicious morning meal, no need to worry. Just take a few minutes the night before to prepare these ingredients in a canning jar and then it heat up a bit the next morning for a sweet, protein- and fiber-rich meal.

1 cup nonfat plain
  Greek yogurt
6 tablespoons almond flour
1 tablespoon chia seeds
1 tablespoon unsweetened
  peanut butter powder
¼ teaspoon stevia
¼ cup diced fresh or frozen
  strawberries

Serving Recommendations
Puree: ¼ to ½ cup

Soft Foods: ½ cup to 1 cup

General: 1 full serving
(about 1 cup)

1. In a pint-size canning jar, mix the yogurt, almond flour, chia seeds, peanut butter powder, and stevia. Set aside.

2. Heat a small skillet over medium heat. Place the strawberries in the skillet. Cook on medium heat for 1 to 2 minutes until the strawberries soften.

3. Pour the strawberries into the jar and mix well with other ingredients. Seal the jar tightly and place in the refrigerator. Allow the mixture to sit overnight for at least 8 hours to set.

4. Scoop out ½ cup of the mixture if you're only eating one serving. Enjoy cold or heat in the microwave for about 30 seconds or so to warm before eating.

STORAGE TIP: Store in a microwave-safe container so you can heat it up safely before enjoying. Store refrigerated for up to 3 days.

PER SERVING (½ CUP): Calories: 232; Protein: 19g; Fat: 13g; Carbohydrates: 14g; Fiber: 8g; Sugar: 6g; Sodium: 45mg

Cinnamon Flax-and-Almond Breakfast Cakes

SERVES 4 / PREP TIME: 5 MINUTES / COOK TIME: 20 MINUTES

Pancakes are a sweet start to your morning, but unfortunately, they're also high in carbohydrates and usually topped in sugary syrup. But there's no need to miss out on the fluffy goodness of pancakes with this almond and flax meal recipe for sweet cinnamon breakfast cakes you can top with your favorite sugar-free jam or syrup.

4 tablespoons flax meal

4 tablespoons
  almond flour

4 tablespoons
  unsweetened
  almond milk

2 large eggs

2 teaspoons brown sugar

1 teaspoon ground
  cinnamon

1 teaspoon vanilla extract

¼ teaspoon stevia

Nonstick cooking spray

Serving Recommendations
SOFT FOODS: 1 to
2 small cakes

GENERAL: 2 to 4 cakes
(depending on tolerance and
daily calorie needs)

1. In a large mixing bowl, combine the flax meal, almond flour, almond milk, eggs, brown sugar, cinnamon, vanilla extract, and stevia with a fork or whisk to create a batter.

2. Coat a large skillet with nonstick cooking spray and heat over medium heat.

3. Use a heaping tablespoon of batter to create small round cakes. Cook for 2 to 3 minutes on each side, until golden brown. You will know the cake is ready to flip since little bubbles will start to form on the surface of the cake.

4. Repeat until all batter has been cooked. This recipe should create about 8 small cakes. Remove from the skillet and serve.

STORAGE TIP: Store the batter for 2 to 3 days in the refrigerator before cooking. Once cooked, the cakes stay fresh in an airtight container up to 3 days in the refrigerator or up to 3 months in the freezer.

PER SERVING (2 SMALL CAKES): Calories: 117; Protein: 7g; Fat: 8g; Carbohydrates: 7g; Fiber: 3g; Sugar: 2g; Sodium: 50mg

Coconut-Almond Breakfast Cakes

SERVES 4 / PREP TIME: 5 MINUTES / COOK TIME: 20 MINUTES

Instead of a sugary muffin or cereal, take a little bit of time to make these fluffy and nutty coconut almond breakfast cakes. These dense and slightly sweet breakfast cakes provide a unique flavor in the pancake form you're used to. Top them with your favorite jam or low-sugar syrup or with sliced berries. You can add more protein and a unique flavor by adding a scoop of vanilla unsweetened whey protein powder to this recipe.

Nonstick cooking spray
1 cup almond flour
½ cup unsweetened
   coconut milk
2 large eggs
2 teaspoons vanilla extract
1 teaspoon ground
   cinnamon
1 teaspoon baking powder
½ teaspoon stevia
¼ teaspoon salt

Serving Recommendations
Soft Foods: 1 to 2 cakes

General: 2 cakes (or more depending on calorie needs daily)

1. Spray a large skillet with nonstick cooking spray and heat over medium heat.

2. While the skillet heats, in a medium bowl, combine the almond flour, coconut milk, eggs, vanilla extract, cinnamon, baking powder, stevia, and salt and beat well until combined.

3. Spoon about 2 tablespoons of the ingredient mixture into the skillet. Cook for 1 to 2 minutes each side, or until golden brown.

4. Repeat with the remainder of the batter, making sure each cake is at least an inch apart from the others if cooking multiple cakes at one time.

5. Remove the cakes from the heat and enjoy plain or with your favorite topping.

STORAGE TIP: Place leftover cakes in an airtight container or on a plate covered with plastic wrap. Refrigerate the leftovers and consume within 3 to 4 days. You can reheat the refrigerated cakes in the microwave for about 30 seconds.

PER SERVING (2 CAKES): Calories: 209; Protein: 9g; Fat: 17g; Carbohydrates: 7g; Fiber: 3g; Sugar: 2g; Sodium: 199mg

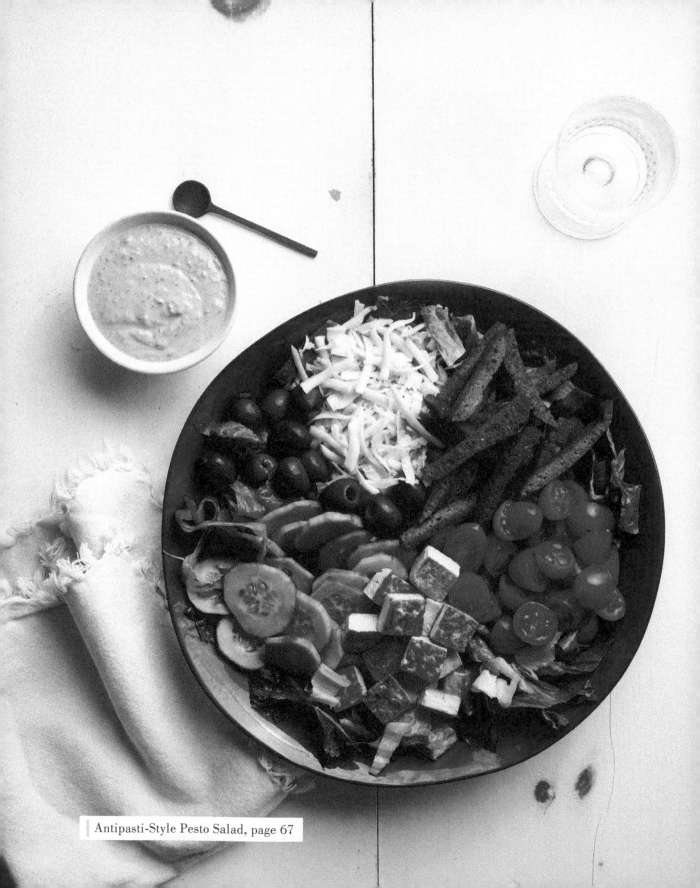

Antipasti-Style Pesto Salad, page 67

Vegetarian

Tofu Scramble

SERVES 4 / PREP TIME: 5 MINUTES / COOK TIME: 10 MINUTES

If you follow a meatless diet and need a break from oats and grains, this recipe will provide the perfect, protein-packed escape. Not only does this recipe resemble the texture and protein content of eggs, but the addition of antioxidant-rich golden turmeric also gives this tofu scramble the look of eggs, too. Pair with fresh fruit or enjoy on sprouted bread for a balanced breakfast.

4 teaspoons extra-virgin olive oil

¼ cup diced yellow onion

12 ounces firm tofu, drained and cut into 1-inch squares

¼ teaspoon ground turmeric

¼ teaspoon garlic powder

¼ teaspoon salt

Freshly ground black pepper *(optional)*

Serving Recommendations

PUREE: ¼ to ½ cup (½ to 1 serving)

SOFT FOODS: ½ cup to 1 cup (1 to 1½ servings)

GENERAL: As tolerated

1. In a medium skillet, heat the oil over medium heat. Add the onion and stir frequently for 5 minutes, or until the onion is translucent.

2. Add the tofu and use a mixing spoon to scramble the tofu into smaller pieces while combining with the onion.

3. Add the turmeric, garlic powder, salt, and pepper (if using) to taste. Continue to stir for 3 to 5 minutes to heat through. Serve warm.

STORAGE TIP: Store leftovers in an airtight container in the refrigerator for up to 3 days.

PER SERVING (½ CUP): Calories: 115; Protein: 7g; Fat: 9g; Carbohydrates: 3g; Fiber: 2g; Sugar: 1g; Sodium: 156mg

Chia Seed and Strawberry Yogurt Parfait

SERVES 1 / PREP TIME: 2 MINUTES / COOK TIME: 5 MINUTES,
PLUS OVERNIGHT CHILLING

This low-carbohydrate yogurt parfait uses chia seeds instead of granola to provide extra fiber and protein to this already protein- and flavor-packed breakfast parfait. Feel free to use other fruits in this parfait, but note that they may add additional carbohydrates to this recipe.

Nonstick cooking spray
½ cup fresh or frozen
   strawberries, sliced
1 cup nonfat plain Greek
   yogurt, divided
¼ teaspoon stevia
   (optional)
1 tablespoon chia
   seeds, divided

Serving Recommendations
PUREE: ¼ to ½ cup (¼ to
½ serving)
SOFT FOODS: ½ cup to 1 cup
(½ to 1 serving)
GENERAL: As tolerated

1. Spray a small skillet with nonstick cooking spray and heat over medium heat. Cook the strawberries for 2 minutes, stirring frequently. Remove from heat.

2. Measure half of the yogurt into a jar or mug and mix in the stevia (if using). Place ½ tablespoon of chia seeds on top, press the chia seeds into the yogurt layer, and top with half of the strawberries. Repeat with a second layer of the remaining yogurt, chia seeds, and berries.

3. Let the mixture set overnight in the refrigerator before serving to give time for the chia seeds to gelatinize. Enjoy chilled.

INGREDIENT TIP: Feel free to use a mixed berry blend if you prefer a variety of flavors in your parfait.

PER SERVING (1¼ TO 1½ CUPS): Calories: 175; Protein: 21g; Fat: 3g; Carbohydrates: 17g; Fiber: 7g; Sugar: 10g; Sodium: 65mg

Vegan Pumpkin Pie–Inspired Overnight No-Oats

SERVES 2 / PREP TIME: 5 MINUTES, PLUS OVERNIGHT CHILLING

If you're rushing around in the morning and end up reaching for a muffin on your way out the door, think again. Opt instead for a delicious and healthy cereal option you can prepare the night before. Consume cold or warmed in the microwave for a hearty breakfast treat. If you don't have high protein plant-based milk on hand (~10 grams per cup) like Silk Protein Almond and Cashew Milk, then create your own by combining 1 cup of unsweetened almond milk and 10 grams of protein worth of unsweetened pea protein powder.

1 cup high-protein
  plant-based milk
6 tablespoons almond flour
1 tablespoon chia seeds
1 teaspoon vanilla extract
1 teaspoon pumpkin
  pie spice
¼ teaspoon stevia
  (optional)

Serving Recommendations
PUREE: ¼ to ½ cup

SOFT FOODS: ½ cup to 1 cup

GENERAL: As tolerated

1. In a pint-size canning jar, combine the protein milk, almond flour, chia seeds, vanilla extract, pumpkin pie spice, and stevia (if using). Seal the jar with a tight-fitting lid and place in the refrigerator. Allow to sit overnight for at least 8 hours to set.

2. Enjoy cold or remove the lid and heat in the microwave for about 30 seconds to warm before eating.

STORAGE TIP: A canning jar with a tightly sealed lid works best for this recipe, especially if you plan on taking the cereal mixture with you on the go. This type of jar, with the lid removed, is also microwave safe. Store for up to 5 days in the refrigerator.

PER SERVING (½ CUP): Calories: 214; Protein: 11g; Fat: 16g; Carbohydrates: 10g; Fiber: 5g; Sugar: 1g; Sodium: 81mg

Butternut Squash Curry Soup

SERVES 4 / PREP TIME: 5 MINUTES / COOK TIME: 10 MINUTES

This butternut squash soup has more spice than your average fall-favorite comfort food. A little bit of garlic and curry powder help spice up this dish and make it a satisfying choice to warm your insides any time of year. If you prefer a less spicy soup, you can add less curry powder. To save time, purchase prepeeled and diced butternut squash cubes and steam in the bag. Typically, a 10-ounce bag of frozen cubes yields about 1 cup cooked cubes.

3 cups peeled and diced butternut squash

1 cup nonfat plain Greek yogurt

1 teaspoon garlic powder

1 teaspoon curry powder

½ teaspoon salt

2 tablespoons pea protein powder (about 33 grams)

1½ cups unsweetened plain almond milk

Serving Recommendation:

PUREE: ¼ to ½ cup (about ½ serving)

SOFT FOODS: ½ cup to 1 cup (about 1 serving)

GENERAL: As tolerated

1. Fill the bottom of a medium saucepan with a couple inches of water and insert a steamer basket. Place the squash in the steamer basket, bring the water to a boil, cover, and steam for 7 to 8 minutes, until softened. Remove from the heat.

2. In a medium bowl, combine the squash, yogurt, garlic powder, curry powder, and salt.

3. In a separate small bowl, mix together the protein powder and almond milk. Then add to the squash and mix well.

4. Place the mixture in a blender and blend on low for 30 to 60 seconds. Pour into bowls and enjoy.

STORAGE TIP: Store in an airtight container in the refrigerator for up to 7 days.

PER SERVING (¾ CUP): Calories: 100; Protein: 12g; Fat: 2g; Carbohydrates: 10g; Fiber: 2g; Sugar: 3g; Sodium: 432mg

Tofu Caesar Salad

SERVES 4 / PREP TIME: 10 MINUTES / COOK TIME: 5 MINUTES

Caesar salad is a favorite of mine, but unfortunately, it's full of excess calories and fat. This tofu Caesar salad uses mozzarella-crusted tofu cubes and Greek yogurt-based Caesar-style dressing. If you prefer croutons with your salad, make the Savory Cheese Biscuits (page 144) and cut them into cubes.

For the dressing
½ cup nonfat plain
  Greek yogurt
½ cup shredded
  Parmesan cheese
Juice of 1 small lemon
  (2 tablespoons)
1 tablespoon extra-virgin
  olive oil
1 teaspoon garlic powder
¼ teaspoon salt
Dash freshly ground
  black pepper

For the salad
2 tablespoons cornstarch
6 tablespoons shredded
  mozzarella cheese
Dash salt
8 ounces firm tofu (1 cup),
  cut into 1-inch cubes
1 tablespoon extra-virgin
  olive oil
2 cups shredded
  romaine lettuce

To make the dressing

1. Add the yogurt, Parmesan cheese, lemon juice, oil, garlic powder, salt, and pepper to a blender or food processor and blend on low for about 30 seconds or until smooth. Set aside.

To make the salad

2. On a plate, mix the cornstarch, mozzarella cheese, and salt. Coat each piece of tofu well with the mixture.

3. Heat the oil in a skillet over medium heat. Sear the tofu for 30 seconds on all sides. Remove the tofu from the heat once all sides are golden brown.

4. Prepare a large bowl with romaine lettuce on the bottom and arrange the tofu on top.

5. Drizzle the dressing on top of the salad and enjoy.

STORAGE TIP: Store the salad and dressing separately in airtight containers for up to 3 days.

Serving Recommendations
PUREE: about ½ serving of tofu and dressing (no lettuce)
SOFT FOODS: ½ cup to 1 cup (1 to 1½ servings of tofu and dressing; no lettuce)

GENERAL: 1 to 2 servings, or more as tolerated

PER SERVING (2 OUNCES OF TOFU, ½ CUP LETTUCE GREENS + 2 TABLESPOONS DRESSING): Calories: 196; Protein: 15g; Fat: 12g; Carbohydrates: 10g; Fiber: 2g; Sugar: 1g; Sodium: 483mg

Antipasti-Style Pesto Salad

SERVES 4 / PREP TIME: 10 MINUTES / COOK TIME: 10 MINUTES

This simple salad is easy to prepare but is full of flavor and can be enjoyed as an entrée or as a starter. This salad can also be converted to a vegan dish if you replace the cheese with vegan cheese alternatives, but note that this will likely change the carbohydrate and fat content.

For the salad
Nonstick cooking spray
4 ounces firm tofu
Dash salt
4 ounces seitan strips
  or slices
2 cups shredded
  romaine lettuce
1 cup shredded
  mozzarella cheese
1 cup halved grape
  tomatoes
1 cup peeled and sliced
  cucumber
12 pitted whole green or
  black olives

For the sauce
1 cup nonfat plain
  Greek yogurt
4 tablespoons pesto sauce

Serving Recommendation:
SOFT FOODS: ½ cup to 1 cup (about 1 serving of protein and soft vegetables without lettuce)

GENERAL: 1 to 2 servings, as tolerated

To make the salad

1. Spray a medium skillet with nonstick cooking spray and heat over medium heat.

2. Sprinkle the tofu with salt and sear for 1 minute on each side, until golden brown. Remove from the heat, dice into cubes, and set aside.

3. Spray the skillet with another coat of cooking spray and heat the seitan for 1 minute on each side. Remove the seitan from the skillet and cut into strips. Set aside.

4. Prepare a large bowl with romaine lettuce on the bottom and arrange the tofu, seitan, mozzarella cheese, tomatoes, cucumber, and olives in separate sections on top of the lettuce.

To make the sauce

5. In a small bowl or mug, combine the Greek yogurt and pesto and mix well.

6. Drizzle the dressing on top of the salad and enjoy.

> **STORAGE TIP:** Store the salad and dressing separately in airtight containers for up to 3 days.

PER SERVING (1 OUNCE EACH OF CHEESE, TOFU, AND SEITAN + 1 CUP VEGETABLES + 5 TABLESPOONS DRESSING): Calories: 279; Protein: 25g; Fat: 16g; Carbohydrates: 10g; Fiber: 3g; Sugar: 3g; Sodium: 559mg

Portobello Mushroom and Broccoli Tempeh Bowl ·

SERVES 5 / PREP TIME: 5 MINUTES / COOK TIME: 20 MINUTES

Tired of tofu? Burnt out on beans? This protein-packed, plant-based bowl is for you. Just a simple combination of cumin, vegetable broth, salt, and cilantro gives this dish a touch of flavor without overpowering the natural umami flavor of the mushrooms and the mildly nutty flavor of the tempeh. Feel free to add more nonstarchy vegetables to this dish like spinach, diced onion, diced peppers, or more broccoli to volumize the dish.

8 ounces tempeh (1⅓ cups)

½ cup water

4 ounces portobello mushroom, sliced in strips (1 to 2 mushrooms)

2 cups chopped broccoli florets

½ cup vegetable broth

1 tablespoon extra-virgin olive oil

¼ teaspoon dried cilantro

¼ teaspoon ground cumin

⅛ teaspoon salt

1. In a small skillet, cook the tempeh and water over medium heat for 8 to 10 minutes to soften. Remove from the skillet and set aside. Discard the water.

2. While the tempeh cooks, in a large skillet, combine the mushrooms, broccoli, and broth over medium heat. Cover and steam the vegetables for 8 to 10 minutes, until tender.

3. Once the broth has mostly evaporated, add the tempeh and oil. Mash the tempeh into small morsels and stir the vegetables and tempeh frequently while cooking for 10 minutes. Add the cilantro, cumin, and salt. Stir well and enjoy warm.

Serving Recommendations
SOFT FOODS: ½ cup to 1 cup (about 1 serving)

GENERAL: As tolerated

STORAGE TIP: Store leftovers in an airtight container in the refrigerator for up to 3 days.

PER SERVING (½ CUP): Calories: 114; Protein: 9g; Fat: 6g; Carbohydrates: 8g; Fiber: 3g; Sugar: 1g; Sodium: 154mg

Tempeh Stir-Fry Bowl with Creamy Peanut Sauce

SERVES 5 / PREP TIME: 5 MINUTES / COOK TIME: 10 MINUTES

If you enjoy the texture of rice and the flavor of Thai-style peanut sauce, you'll love this tempeh stir-fry bowl. A combination of low-carbohydrate vegetables, soy sauce, tempeh, and homemade peanut sauce gives this dish a unique flavor, while providing plenty of the protein that you need.

8 ounces tempeh

½ cup water

1 tablespoon extra-virgin olive oil

1 cup sliced zucchini

½ cup chopped yellow onion

½ cup peeled, thinly sliced carrot

1 teaspoon soy sauce

1 recipe Creamy Peanut Sauce (page 164)

Serving Recommendations

SOFT FOODS: ½ cup to 1 cup (½ to 1 serving)

GENERAL: 1 to 2 servings, or more as tolerated

1. In a small skillet, combine the tempeh and water. Cook on medium heat for 8 minutes, until softened. Remove from the skillet and set aside. Discard the water.

2. While the tempeh cooks, heat the oil in a large skillet over medium heat. Add the zucchini, onion, and carrot. Cook for 8 minutes, stirring frequently, or until the onion is translucent and the carrot can be cut in half easily with a spatula or fork. Stir in the soy sauce and toss well.

3. Serve the vegetables over the tempeh and drizzle the peanut sauce on top. Toss to coat well and enjoy.

STORAGE TIP: Store leftovers in an airtight container in the refrigerator for up to 3 days.

PER SERVING (¾ STIR-FRY + 3 TABLESPOONS SAUCE): Calories: 261; Protein: 18g; Fat: 15g; Carbohydrates: 16g; Fiber: 5g; Sugar: 5g; Sodium: 405mg

Tempeh-and-Parmesan Risotto

SERVES 5 / PREP TIME: 5 MINUTES / COOK TIME: 35 MINUTES

Tempeh doesn't have to be off-limits on a soft food diet, and it doesn't have to be bland. Simmered in nonfat Greek yogurt and cheese, this meatless dish can take on the flavor and texture of creamy risotto. Feel free to add additional unsweetened soy milk if you prefer a thinner consistency.

8 ounces tempeh
½ cup water
½ cup diced onion
1 tablespoon
   unsalted butter
¼ teaspoon salt
1 cup unsweetened soymilk
½ cup nonfat plain
   Greek yogurt
1 cup shredded
   Parmesan cheese

Serving Recommendations
SOFT FOODS: ½ cup to 1 cup (about 1 serving)
GENERAL: As tolerated

1. In a medium saucepan, combine the tempeh and water and cook on medium heat for about 8 minutes, until softened.

2. Add the onion, butter, and salt and cook for 5 to 7 minutes, or until the onion is translucent.

3. Add the soymilk and yogurt to the pan. Bring to a rolling boil. Fold in the Parmesan cheese and cook for another 15 to 20 minutes on low-to-medium heat or until sauce thickens, stirring frequently. Remove from heat and serve.

COOKING TIP: Cook time may vary depending on your heat source. Gas stoves may cook faster than the listed time, whereas electric stove tops may cook slower. It's best to supervise the dish and just make sure the sauce is at a rolling boil during cooking; if not boiling after several minutes, then bring heat up a bit to medium and continue cooking until sauce thickens.

STORAGE TIP: Store leftovers in an airtight container in the refrigerator for up to 3 days.

PER SERVING (½ CUP): Calories: 243; Protein: 21g; Fat: 15g; Carbohydrates: 8g; Fiber: 2g; Sugar: 1g; Sodium: 466mg

Tofu Burgers

SERVES 4 / PREP TIME: 5 MINUTES / COOK TIME: 15 MINUTES

Enjoy the protein-packed goodness of burgers without the fat and sodium. Unlike many tofu burger recipes, this meatless patty is free of starchy fillers like wheat flour or beans and, if you follow an egg-free regimen, can be modified by using a chia seeds. One egg equals 1 tablespoon chia seeds mixed with 3 tablespoons water. Let the mixture sit at room temperature for 30 minutes before using.

1 tablespoon extra-virgin olive oil

½ cup diced yellow onion

8 ounces firm tofu, drained well

4 tablespoons almond flour

1 large egg

2 teaspoons garlic powder

¼ teaspoon salt

Nonstick cooking spray

Serving Recommendations
SOFT FOODS: ½ cup to 1 cup (about 1 to 1½ burgers)
GENERAL: As tolerated

1. In a large skillet, heat the oil over medium heat. Add the onion and cook, stirring frequently, for 5 minutes or until the onion is translucent.

2. In a large mixing bowl, combine the onion, tofu, almond flour, egg, garlic powder, and salt with a fork, making sure to mash the tofu well and combine the egg with all ingredients.

3. Spray a skillet with cooking spray and heat over medium heat.

4. Split mixture into 8 small burger patties (you may have to cook multiple batches depending on how big your skillet is). Make sure burgers are an inch apart from each other to allow for flipping.

5. Cook the burgers for about 5 minutes on each side. Before flipping burgers, spray the top side with cooking spray to prevent sticking to the skillet. Remove from the heat and serve alone, on a lettuce wrap, or on your favorite whole-grain bread or wrap.

STORAGE TIP: Store leftovers in an airtight container in the refrigerator for up to 5 days.

PER SERVING (2 SMALL BURGERS): Calories: 148; Protein: 8g; Fat: 11g; Carbohydrates: 6g; Fiber: 3g; Sugar: 1g; Sodium: 172mg

Zucchini Noodles and Meatless Meat Sauce

SERVES 5 / PREP TIME: 5 MINUTES / COOK TIME: 30 MINUTES

Try spicing up soy protein with this "meat" sauce recipe for your low-carbohydrate pasta alternative. The zucchini adds the texture of pasta without all the carbohydrates, while the soy protein meat sauce provides the savory flavor of standard Bolognese while still maintaining the protein content.

For the zucchini noodles

1 tablespoon extra-virgin olive oil

2 medium zucchini, peeled and spiralized

For the "meat" sauce

1 tablespoon extra-virgin olive oil

1 cup soy protein crumbles

1 cup diced yellow onion

2 cups chopped tomato

2 teaspoons garlic powder

2 teaspoons Italian seasoning

¼ teaspoon salt

1 cup shredded mozzarella cheese

Serving Recommendation

Soft Foods: ½ cup to 1 cup (about 1 serving)

General: As tolerated

To make the zucchini noodles

1. In a large skillet, heat the oil over medium heat.

2. Place the zucchini in the skillet and cook, stirring every 30 seconds or so, for 4 to 6 minutes, until softened. Remove from the heat and place the zucchini in serving bowl.

To make the "meat" sauce

3. In the same skillet, heat the oil over medium. Add the soy protein crumbles and cook for 5 to 7 minutes. Add the onion and cook for 5 to 7 minutes, stirring frequently, or until translucent.

4. Add the tomato, garlic powder, Italian seasoning, and salt and mix well. Reduce the heat to medium-low and simmer for 7 to 10 minutes, stirring regularly, until the sauce thickens.

5. Remove from the heat and pour the sauce over zucchini noodles. Top with mozzarella cheese before serving.

> **STORAGE TIP:** Store the leftover sauce and zucchini noodles separately in airtight containers in the refrigerator for up to 5 days.

PER SERVING (¾ CUP ZUCCHINI NOODLES + ¾ CUP SAUCE):
Calories: 217; Protein: 15g; Fat: 13g; Carbohydrates: 11g; Fiber: 4g; Sugar: 4g; Sodium: 435mg

Zucchini Noodles with Vegan Garlic Cream Sauce

SERVES 5 / PREP TIME: 5 MINUTES / COOK TIME: 10 MINUTES

If you love spaghetti but are trying to cut down on carbohydrates, zucchini noodles are a healthy and easy alternative. And if you don't eat dairy or are trying to cut back on fat, you'll love this alfredo-esque creamy garlic sauce made from blended tofu and garlic. This recipe checks all the boxes for flavor, fiber, and protein-packed deliciousness. If you don't have a spiralizer, you can use a vegetable peeler to peel thin strips of the zucchini.

2 tablespoons extra-virgin
   olive oil
5 medium zucchinis,
   peeled and spiralized
1 recipe Vegan Garlic
   Cream Sauce (page 162)

Serving Recommendations
Soft Foods: ½ cup to 1 cup (about 1 serving)
General: As tolerated

1. In a large skillet, heat the oil over medium heat.

2. Place the zucchini in the skillet and cook, stirring every 30 seconds or so with a fork or tongs, for 4 to 6 minutes, until softened. Remove from the heat and place the zucchini in serving bowl or on a plate.

3. In the same skillet, warm the garlic cream sauce over low heat for 1 to 3 minutes.

4. Serve over the zucchini noodles and use tongs or a fork to lightly coat zucchini noodles with sauce before serving.

> **STORAGE TIP:** Store the zucchini noodles and sauce in separate airtight containers and combine before reheating and serving. Store refrigerated for up to 5 days.

PER SERVING (¾ CUP ZUCCHINI NOODLES + ¼ CUP SAUCE):
Calories: 75; Protein: 5g; Fat: 12g; Carbohydrates: 8g; Fiber: 3g; Sugar: 4g; Sodium: 130mg

Barbecue Jackfruit Biscuit with Zucchini-Yogurt Spread

SERVES 4 / PREP TIME: 10 MINUTES / COOK TIME: 25 MINUTES

If you love pulled pork, you'll love this vegetarian-friendly barbecue jackfruit sandwich biscuit. This creation uses Savory Cheese Biscuits (page 144) and tops them with flavorful shredded jackfruit balanced with refreshing homemade zucchini-yogurt spread. For your sugar-free barbecue choice, I recommend either Stubb's or G. Hughes brands.

For the jackfruit
Nonstick cooking spray
½ cup sliced canned jackfruit, drained
¼ cup water
1 tablespoon sugar-free barbecue sauce
½ teaspoon brown sugar

For the spread
Nonstick cooking spray
1 cup peeled, diced zucchini
4 tablespoons nonfat plain Greek yogurt
¼ teaspoon garlic powder
⅛ teaspoon salt
½ recipe Savory Cheese Biscuits (page 144)

Serving Recommendation:
SOFT FOODS: ½ cup to 1 cup (about 1 biscuit)

GENERAL: 1 full serving or more as tolerated

To make the jackfruit

1. Spray a medium skillet with nonstick cooking spray and then place over medium heat. Add the jackfruit and cook for about 5 minutes, stirring frequently as the jackfruit softens. Add the water.

2. Cook for another 5 minutes, or until the water is absorbed and the jackfruit is softened, stirring frequently. Remove from the heat.

3. Place the jackfruit in a medium mixing bowl and use a fork to shred it into small pieces. Add in the barbecue sauce and brown sugar while stirring.

To make the spread

4. Coat the same skillet well with cooking spray and heat over medium heat. Cook the zucchini, stirring occasionally, for 10 to 12 minutes, until softened and slightly golden brown on each side.

5. Remove the zucchini from the skillet and transfer to a blender or food processor with the yogurt, garlic powder, and salt. Blend for 30 to 60 seconds or until smooth.

6. Split each biscuit in half. Spread 1 tablespoon of the spread on one side of a biscuit. Scoop 1 tablespoon of the jackfruit mixture onto the other side of the biscuit. Repeat with the remaining ingredients, then top the jackfruit biscuit halves with the zucchini-yogurt spread biscuit halves to make 4 biscuit sandwiches.

STORAGE TIP: If you have leftovers, you should store each ingredient (biscuit, jackfruit, and spread) separately. Keep biscuits in a dry, cool place, like in a plastic storage bag in your pantry for up to 3 days. The spread and jackfruit can be stored in separate airtight containers in the refrigerator for up to 7 days.

PER SERVING (2 BISCUITS + 2 TABLESPOONS JACKFRUIT + 1 TABLESPOON SPREAD): Calories: 311; Protein: 17g; Fat: 23g; Carbohydrates: 16g; Fiber: 4g; Sugar: 7g; Sodium: 532mg

Vegetarian Chili

SERVES 5 / PREP TIME: 10 MINUTES / COOK TIME: 40 MINUTES

A hot bowl of chili can warm you inside and out. This filling dish of protein and vegetables is not just for meat eaters but can be just as satisfying and flavorful in its plant-based form. Find soy protein crumbles in the frozen or vegetarian foods section of your grocery store. For more protein, you can add a dollop of plain Greek yogurt to act as a sour cream alternative. Feel free to add other nonstarchy vegetables such as diced bell pepper, garlic, or other peppers to taste.

1 tablespoon extra-virgin olive oil

1 cup chopped yellow onion

1 cup canned diced tomatoes

½ cup shelled edamame

1 teaspoon dried cilantro

1 teaspoon chili powder

1 teaspoon ground cumin

¼ teaspoon salt

1 cup meatless soy protein crumbles

1 cup of water

8 tablespoons shredded Cheddar cheese

1. In a medium saucepan, heat the oil over medium heat. Cook the onion for 5 to 7 minutes, stirring frequently, until it is translucent.

2. Add in the tomatoes and their juices, edamame, cilantro, chili powder, cumin, and salt. Cook for about 10 minutes.

3. Add the soy protein crumbles and water to the pan and cook for another 10 minutes.

4. Simmer the chili for at least 5 to 10 minutes, until chili thickens.

5. Remove from the heat and top the chili with Cheddar cheese to serve.

STORAGE TIP: Store leftovers in an airtight container in the refrigerator for up to 5 days.

PER SERVING (½ CUP OF CHILI + 2 TABLESPOONS CHEESE):
Calories: 134; Protein: 10g; Fat: 7g; Carbohydrates: 9g; Fiber: 3g; Sugar: 3g; Sodium: 351mg

Serving Recommendations

PUREE: ¼ to ½ cup (about ½ serving; blend chili in blender before serving)

SOFT FOODS: ½ cup to 1 cup (about 1 serving)

GENERAL: As tolerated

Parmesan-Crusted Scallops and Greens, page 90

Fish and Seafood

Shrimp Gazpacho-Style Soup

SERVES 4 / PREP TIME: 10 MINUTES / COOK TIME: 10 MINUTES

Tired of the same old tomato soup? If so, add a bit of shrimp and citrus flavor for a gazpacho-style soup that works great as a refreshing meal starter or lunch. The shrimp provides plenty of protein, while the veggies add colorful antioxidants and fiber. Feel free to add chili pepper or hot sauce to the mixture if you prefer a spicy soup. Enjoy chilled or warm per your preference.

1 tablespoon extra-virgin olive oil

1 cup chopped yellow onion

½ cup diced bell pepper

3 cups chopped tomato

4 teaspoons freshly squeezed lemon juice

½ teaspoon salt

1½ cups cooked shrimp

Serving Recommendations

SOFT FOODS: 1 full serving

GENERAL: 1 to 2 full servings, depending on daily calorie needs

1. Coat a medium skillet with the oil and heat over medium heat. Add the onion and pepper, and cook for 5 to 7 minutes, stirring occasionally, until the onion is slightly translucent.

2. Add the cooked onion and pepper, tomato, lemon juice, and salt to a blender. Blend for 1 to 2 minutes on high or until mixture is smooth.

3. Pour the soup into a bowl and add the shrimp. Enjoy.

STORAGE TIP: Store leftovers in an airtight container in the refrigerator for up to 3 days.

PER SERVING (6 TABLESPOONS SHRIMP + ½ CUP SOUP):
Calories: 109; Protein: 11g; Fat: 4g; Carbohydrates: 9g; Fiber: 3g; Sugar: 7g; Sodium: 484mg

Shrimp Cauliflower Chowder

SERVES 4 / PREP TIME: 10 MINUTES / COOK TIME: 25 MINUTES

Clam chowder is a rich seafood dish infamous for its thick and creamy base. However, its thickness comes from butter, flour, cream, and potatoes, which add lots of fat and carbohydrates. You'll love this low-fat and low-carbohydrate creamy-textured chowder recipe. To save time, use steam-in-the-bag cauliflower rice and microwave while the onion is cooking.

1 tablespoon extra-virgin olive oil

1 cup diced yellow onion

1 cup cauliflower rice

½ cup water

¼ teaspoon salt

½ cup unsweetened light canned coconut milk

½ unsweetened almond milk

4 tablespoons nutritional yeast

Dash freshly ground black pepper

1½ cups peeled raw small salad shrimp

Serving Recommendations

SOFT FOODS: 1 full serving

GENERAL: 1 to 2 full servings, depending on daily calorie needs

1. In a medium saucepan, heat the oil over medium heat. Cook the onion for 5 to 7 minutes, stirring frequently, or until the onion is slightly translucent.

2. Add the cauliflower rice, water, and salt. Cook for 6 to 8 minutes, stirring occasionally, until cauliflower is softened and the water is absorbed.

3. Add the coconut milk, almond milk, nutritional yeast, and pepper to the pot and stir well. Simmer on low-to-medium heat for 1 to 2 minutes. Remove from heat.

4. Pour the mixture into a blender and blend for 1 to 2 minutes on low until the mixture is smooth.

5. Pour the mixture back into the pot and add the shrimp. Simmer on low to medium heat for 5 to 7 minutes, until the shrimp are pink and cooked through. Remove from heat and serve.

STORAGE TIP: Store leftovers in an airtight container in the refrigerator for up to 3 days.

PER SERVING (6 TABLESPOONS SHRIMP + ½ CUP CHOWDER):
Calories: 133; Protein: 14g; Fat: 6g; Carbohydrates: 6g; Fiber: 3g; Sugar: 3g; Sodium: 358mg

Shrimp Toast–Style Low-Carb Seafood Cakes

MAKES 8 / PREP TIME: 5 MINUTES / COOK TIME: 15 MINUTES

If you've gotten Chinese takeout before, chances are you've tried shrimp toast. This crispy appetizer is basically toast stuffed with savory shrimp filling and fried to a golden-brown crisp. But if you're trying to limit fat, it's off-limits These mini shrimp toast–style cakes will give you the same flavor with less fat and calories.

½ cup canned baby shrimp

4 tablespoons almond flour

2 tablespoons coconut aminos, plus more for dipping

2 tablespoons unsweetened almond milk

2 tablespoons light unsweetened canned coconut milk

1 large egg

½ teaspoon garlic powder

½ teaspoon ginger powder

½ teaspoon chopped parsley or dried

¼ teaspoon salt

1 tablespoon extra-virgin olive oil

⅓ cup finely diced yellow onion

Nonstick cooking spray (optional)

1. In a large mixing bowl, combine the shrimp, almond flour, coconut aminos, almond milk, coconut milk, egg, garlic powder, ginger powder, parsley, and salt. Mix well and set aside.

2. In a medium skillet, heat the oil over medium heat. Cook the onion for about 5 minutes or until slightly translucent. Remove from the heat and add to the shrimp mixture. Incorporate well.

3. Scoop a heaping tablespoon or two of the shrimp mixture into the same skillet and flatten with the back of a spoon. Repeat with the remaining shrimp mixture to make 8 cakes.

4. Cook the shrimp cakes for 3 to 4 minutes on each side, or until each side is a little more than golden brown, working in batches if needed. If the cakes stick to the skillet, spray lightly with cooking spray to prevent sticking.

5. Remove the cakes from the heat and enjoy with additional coconut aminos on the side for dipping.

> **STORAGE TIP:** Store leftovers in an airtight container in the refrigerator for up to 3 days.

Serving Recommendations

SOFT FOODS: 2 to 4 mini cakes

GENERAL: 4 mini cakes, or more depending on daily calorie needs

---

PER SERVING (2 CAKES): Calories: 124; Protein: 7g; Fat: 9g; Carbohydrates: 5g; Fiber: 1g; Sugar: 2g; Sodium: 445mg

Roasted Vegetable and Shrimp Salad

SERVES 4 / PREP TIME: 5 MINUTES / COOK TIME: 20 MINUTES

Add roasted vegetables to your typical shrimp salad for a refreshing take on this protein-rich lunch dish. With a dollop of Greek yogurt instead of mayonnaise, you can significantly reduce the fat compared to other shrimp salad recipes. Feel free to add more Greek yogurt if you prefer a creamier shrimp salad, but you may have to add extra spices to achieve a similar flavor.

Nonstick cooking spray

¼ cup diced yellow or
  red onion

¼ cup diced bell pepper

2 teaspoons extra-virgin
  olive oil, divided

1½ cups canned
  baby shrimp

2 tablespoons nonfat plain
  Greek yogurt

1 teaspoon apple
  cider vinegar

½ teaspoon garlic powder

½ teaspoon ground cumin

Serving Recommendations

SOFT FOODS: 1 serving
(about ½ cup salad)

GENERAL: 1 to 2 servings
(½ to 1 cup salad)

1. Preheat the oven to 400°F. Line a baking sheet with parchment paper or aluminum foil and spray with nonstick cooking spray.

2. Arrange the onion and pepper on the baking sheet and drizzle with 1 tablespoon of oil. Toss the vegetables with the oil and coat well. Bake for about 20 minutes, until all the vegetables are softened and lightly browned. Remove from heat.

3. In a large mixing bowl, combine the onion and pepper with the shrimp, yogurt, remaining oil, vinegar, garlic powder, and cumin.

4. Serve warm or chill in the refrigerator before serving.

STORAGE TIP: Store leftovers in an airtight container in the refrigerator for up to 3 days.

PER SERVING (½ CUP): Calories: 71; Protein: 10g; Fat: 3g; Carbohydrates: 2g; Fiber: <1g; Sugar: 1g; Sodium: 189mg

Coconut-Crusted Shrimp with Simple Cucumber Salad

SERVES 4 / PREP TIME: 10 MINUTES / COOK TIME: 15 MINUTES

Coconut shrimp is typically high in fat and carbohydrates. But this coconut-crusted shrimp recipe brings the flavor with fewer carbohydrates and calories, so you can enjoy it any time. If you prefer a crispier, more golden-brown crust on your shrimp, brush the battered shrimp with olive oil before cooking.

1 tablespoon cornstarch or rice flour

½ teaspoon ginger powder

⅛ teaspoon salt

3 tablespoons coconut flour

1 large egg

1 pound large raw shrimp, shelled and deveined

1 cup cucumber, diced (about 1 small cucumber)

1 tablespoon white rice vinegar

Dash ground black pepper

Dash salt

Serving Recommendations

SOFT FOODS: 1 full serving

GENERAL: 1 to 2 full servings, depending on daily calorie needs

1. Preheat the oven to 400°F. Line a baking sheet with parchment paper and set aside.

2. Prepare two plates, one with cornstarch, ginger, and salt mixed well and the other with coconut flour. Beat the egg in a small bowl and place it between the plates.

3. Take each piece of shrimp and coat lightly on all sides with the cornstarch mixture. Then, coat it completely in egg before coating well with the coconut flour. Place the battered shrimp on the prepared baking sheet.

4. Bake the shrimp for 12 to 14 minutes, or until the batter is golden brown. Flip the shrimp with tongs halfway through cooking.

5. In a medium mixing bowl, combine the cucumber, rice vinegar, pepper, and salt.

6. Serve the shrimp with a side of cucumber salad.

> **STORAGE TIP:** Shrimp are best when freshly cooked and crisp. Store the leftover cucumber salad in an airtight container in the refrigerator for up to 7 days.

PER SERVING (6 SHRIMP + ¼ CUP CUCUMBER SALAD): Calories: 95; Protein: 11g; Fat: 3g; Carbohydrates: 7g; Fiber: 2g; Sugar: 1g; Sodium: 460mg

Broccoli and Garlic Shrimp Stir-Fry

SERVES 4 / PREP TIME: 10 MINUTES / COOK TIME: 25 MINUTES

When you need a break from meat but still want a savory flavor, this stir-fry option is just what you're looking for. The garlic and onion flavors provide just the right amount of potency without overpowering the light protein profile of the shrimp. Pair with more vegetables or a protein- and fiber-rich grain like quinoa for a filling meal option.

2 pounds raw shrimp, deveined

1 tablespoon extra-virgin olive oil

1 cup diced yellow onion

1 medium bell pepper, diced

2 cups chopped broccoli florets

1 teaspoon garlic powder

¼ teaspoon salt

½ cup water

Serving Recommendations
GENERAL: 1 full serving

1. In a large pot, bring a large amount of water to a boil. When the water is boiling, add the shrimp. Cover and reduce the heat to medium. Cook for 5 minutes, or until shrimp turn pink. Remove from the heat, drain the water, and add cold water to the pot. Let the shrimp sit in the cold water for about 5 minutes.

2. Drain the water and peel the shrimp. Place the peeled shrimp in a large bowl and set aside.

3. Coat a large skillet with the oil and heat over medium-high heat. Add the onion and bell pepper. Cook for 5 minutes, or until the onion is translucent and the pepper is softened slightly.

4. Add the broccoli, garlic powder, salt, and ½ cup water. Cover and cook for 5 to 7 minutes, or until the broccoli is cooked slightly.

5. Add in the steamed shrimp and stir frequently for 2 to 3 minutes until all ingredients are combined. Enjoy warm.

STORAGE TIP: Store leftovers in an airtight container in the refrigerator for up to 3 days.

PER SERVING (12 SHRIMP + 1 CUP VEGETABLES): Calories: 235; Protein: 35g; Fat: 4g; Carbohydrates: 10g; Fiber: 3g; Sugar: 4g; Sodium: 166mg

Garlic Pepper Scallops with Broccoli

SERVES 4 / PREP TIME: 5 MINUTES / COOK TIME: 10 MINUTES

If you prefer seafood but are tired of eating fish, scallops are a healthy and delicious alternative full of protein. Just a simple garlic pepper rub and a side of broccoli can make this seafood dish flavorful and filling. And the best part is that this entire meal only takes about 10 minutes to make, so you can enjoy it even on your busiest days.

1 pound raw jumbo sea scallops

1 tablespoon garlic powder

½ teaspoon freshly ground black pepper

⅛ teaspoon salt

2 tablespoons extra-virgin olive oil

2 cups chopped broccoli florets

¼ cup water

Serving Recommendations
GENERAL: 1 full serving

1. Blot the scallops dry with a paper towel.

2. In a small bowl, mix the garlic powder, pepper, and salt and set aside.

3. Coat a large skillet with the oil and heat over medium-high heat.

4. One at a time, lightly dab each scallop with the spice mixture on both flat sides. Place the scallop in the skillet. Repeat with remaining scallops.

5. Cook the scallops for 2 minutes on each side. Remove the scallops to a plate and set aside.

6. Lower the heat to medium and place the broccoli in the skillet. Add the water, cover, and steam for 3 to 5 minutes, or until the broccoli is tender. Drain the broccoli and sprinkle with salt and pepper to taste.

7. Serve the scallops over the broccoli.

> **STORAGE TIP:** Store leftovers in an airtight container in the refrigerator for up to 3 days.

PER SERVING (3 OR 4 SCALLOPS + ½ CUP BROCCOLI):
Calories: 164; Protein: 9g; Fat: 8g; Carbohydrates: 8g; Fiber: 1g; Sugar: 1g; Sodium: 236mg

Almond-Crusted Cod and Roasted Carrots

SERVES 4 / PREP TIME: 10 MINUTES / COOK TIME: 45 MINUTES

If you enjoy fish and chips, but you don't enjoy the extra fat and calories that come with it, there's no need to nix it from your diet forever. This recipe coats cod in a nutty almond flour mixture that bakes to a flavorful batter. And you won't miss the chips once you've tried this simple-but-delicious roasted carrots recipe.

Nonstick cooking spray
1 pound cod fillets
   (4 ounces each)
½ cup almond flour
3 tablespoons cornstarch
¼ teaspoon salt
Freshly ground
   black pepper
2 large eggs
3 medium carrots, peeled

Serving Recommendations
SOFT: ½ to 1 full serving
GENERAL: 1 full serving

1. Preheat the oven to 400°F. Line a baking sheet with parchment paper and spray lightly with cooking spray. Set aside.

2. Blot the cod dry with paper towels and slice into 4-ounce pieces. Set aside.

3. Place the almond flour on a medium plate. On another plate, combine the cornstarch, salt, and pepper. Crack the eggs into a small bowl and beat well.

4. Dip to coat each piece of cod in the cornstarch and salt mixture, then the egg, and then coat well with the almond flour. Place each coated fish piece on the lined baking sheet and repeat for other remaining cod pieces. Set aside.

5. Slice the carrots into ½-inch-thick and 4-inch-long French fry–like pieces and place on the baking sheet next to the cod.

6. Bake for 25 to 30 minutes, flipping the carrots and fish halfway through the cooking time, or when the batter on the fish is golden brown. After 30 minutes, use a large spatula to remove the fish from the baking sheet and set aside.

7. Continue to bake the carrots for another 15 minutes, until browned and tender. Remove from the heat and serve the cod and carrots together.

STORAGE TIP: This is best if consumed fresh to enjoy the crispy crust of the fish, but leftovers of the fish can be stored in an airtight container for up to 3 days. Store the carrots separately in an airtight container for up to 7 days.

PER SERVING (3 TABLESPOONS): Calories: 270; Protein: 33g; Fat: 11g; Carbohydrates: 14g; Fiber: 3g; Sugar: 4g; Sodium: 395mg

Parmesan-Crusted Scallops and Greens

SERVES 4 / PREP TIME: 5 MINUTES / COOK TIME: 15 MINUTES

Add more flavor to your seafood meal with a bit of cheese. You don't need much to create a crispy and flavorful crust on your scallops. When paired with greens, this recipe can provide a balanced meal of healthy protein and antioxidant-rich leafy greens that can be prepared in less than 15 minutes.

1 pound raw jumbo sea scallops

¼ cup cornstarch

1 large egg

½ cup grated Parmesan cheese

½ teaspoon dried or chopped fresh parsley

2 tablespoons extra-virgin olive oil

2 cups baby spinach leaves

Salt

Freshly ground black pepper

Serving Recommendations
SOFT: ½ to 1 full serving
GENERAL: 1 full serving

1. Blot the scallops dry with a paper towel. Leave a bit of moisture on the scallops so the cornstarch will stick, but not too much or the batter will not adhere as well.

2. Place the cornstarch in one small bowl. Beat an egg in another small bowl. Combine the Parmesan cheese and parsley on a medium plate.

3. In a medium skillet, heat the oil over medium heat.

4. One at a time, lightly coat each scallop with cornstarch on both flat sides, dip both sides in the egg, and then coat in the cheese and parsley mixture and set aside. Repeat for all scallops, then place the scallops in the hot skillet. Cook for 3 to 4 minutes on each side until golden brown. Remove from heat and set aside.

5. Lower heat to medium and place the spinach in the skillet. Cook for 3 to 5 minutes or until spinach is wilted. Sprinkle with salt and pepper to taste.

6. Serve the scallops over the spinach.

STORAGE TIP: This is best when consumed fresh but leftovers can be stored in an airtight container for up to 3 days.

PER SERVING (3 TO 4 SCALLOPS + ½ CUP SPINACH): Calories: 248; Protein: 24g; Fat: 12g; Carbohydrates: 12g; Fiber: 1g; Sugar: 0g; Sodium: 406mg

Lemon-Dill Cod with Sautéed Veggie Salsa

SERVES 4 / PREP TIME: 5 MINUTES, PLUS 30 MINUTES TO MARINATE / COOK TIME: 10 MINUTES

A squeeze of lemon and a sprinkle of dill and garlic provide just the right amount of seasoning for this pan-cooked cod dish. Pair with a sautéed veggie salsa for a refreshing combination high in protein, antioxidants, and flavor. Feel free to add low-carbohydrate hot sauce or chili pepper sauce for extra flavor if you tolerate spicy foods.

12 ounces cod fillets

Juice of 3 lemons

1 teaspoon garlic powder

1 teaspoon dillweed

Dash freshly ground
   black pepper

1 tablespoon extra-virgin
   olive oil

1 cup peeled, diced
   zucchini

½ cup canned diced
   tomatoes, drained

½ cup diced sweet
   yellow onion

Serving Recommendations

SOFT: ½ serving

GENERAL: 1 full serving

1. In a shallow, medium casserole dish, place the fish fillets and squeeze the lemon juice on top.

2. In a small bowl, combine the garlic powder and dillweed. Rub each fish fillet with the mixture. Sprinkle the pepper on top of the fish. Place in the refrigerator to marinate for 30 minutes.

3. In a medium skillet, heat the oil over medium heat. Place the fish in center of skillet and the zucchini, tomatoes, and onion on the exterior. Cook the fish for 3 to 4 minutes on each side while stirring the vegetables, until the fish flakes easily with a fork and the vegetables are tender.

4. Remove from heat and serve the fish with a side of vegetables.

STORAGE TIP: This dish is best if consumed immediately, but the vegetables and fish can be stored separately in airtight containers in the refrigerator for up to 3 days.

PER SERVING (3 OUNCES COD + ½ CUP VEGETABLES): Calories: 119; Protein: 12g; Fat: 6g; Carbohydrates: 7g; Fiber: 1g; Sugar: 4g; Sodium: 402mg

Parmesan-Coated Cod with Diced Tomatoes

SERVES 4 / PREP TIME: 10 MINUTES / COOK TIME: 15 MINUTES

Chicken Parmesan is an Italian classic. But on days when you need a break from chicken, bake up this seafood version of the traditional dish and enjoy with fresh, slightly pan-cooked diced tomatoes. You can also enjoy this recipe with zucchini noodles or spaghetti squash for extra fiber.

4 teaspoons cornstarch
1 teaspoon garlic powder
½ teaspoon Italian seasoning
7 tablespoons almond flour
1 large egg
¾ pound cod fillets
¼ cup shredded Parmesan cheese
2 cups canned diced tomatoes, drained

Serving Recommendations
SOFT FOODS: about 1½ ounces or ¼ cup fish and ¼ cup tomatoes
GENERAL: 1 full serving

1. Preheat the oven to 400°F. Line a baking sheet with parchment paper and set aside.

2. On a medium plate, combine the cornstarch, garlic powder, and Italian seasoning. Place the almond flour on another plate. Beat the egg in a small bowl and place it between the plates.

3. Coat the fish lightly with cornstarch, then coat completely in egg, and then coat well with the almond flour. Place the coated fish on the baking sheet.

4. Sprinkle the Parmesan cheese on top of the fish fillets and bake for 12 to 14 minutes, or until cheese is melted and the fish flakes easily with a fork.

5. While the fish bakes, heat a small skillet on medium. Warm the tomatoes for 2 to 3 minutes.

6. Remove the fish from oven, top with the tomatoes, and enjoy.

> **STORAGE TIP:** This dish is best if consumed fresh, but leftovers of the fish and tomatoes can be stored separately in airtight containers in the refrigerator for up to 3 days.

PER SERVING (3 OUNCES COD + ½ CUP TOMATOES): Calories: 221; Protein: 18.5g; Fat: 12.25g; Carbohydrates: 11.25; Fiber: 2.4g; Sugar: 3.5g; Sodium: 414mg

Fish Taco Bowl with Cauliflower Rice

SERVES 4 / PREP TIME: 10 MINUTES / COOK TIME: 15 MINUTES

Enjoy the fresh flavor of fish tacos without the carbohydrates from the tortilla and the fat from the typically creamy toppings. This fish taco bowl is simple in ingredients and preparation, but rich in flavor as well as protein and fiber. If tolerated, you can enjoy this creation with a lettuce wrap or low-carbohydrate tortilla.

2 cups cauliflower rice

Dash salt

1 tablespoon extra-virgin olive oil

12 ounces cod fillets

½ cup diced red onion

1 cup sliced avocado

1 tablespoon freshly squeezed lemon juice

1 teaspoon dried or chopped fresh cilantro

Serving Recommendations

SOFT FOODS: about ½ serving (about 1½ ounces fish, 1 tablespoon onion, 2 tablespoons avocado, and ¼ cup cauliflower rice)

GENERAL: 1 full serving

1. Fill the bottom of a medium saucepan with a few inches of water and insert a steamer basket. Place the cauliflower rice in the steamer basket, bring the water to a boil, cover, and steam for 7 to 9 minutes, until soft. Remove from the heat, mix in the salt, and set aside.

2. In a large skillet, heat the olive oil over medium heat. Place the fish fillets in the center of the skillet and the red onion on the exterior.

3. Cook the fish for 3 to 4 minutes on each side while stirring the onion during cooking, until the fish flakes with a fork and the onion is softened.

4. Remove from heat. Place the cauliflower rice in a bowl and top with the fish and cooked onions. Top with sliced avocado, lemon juice, and cilantro.

> **STORAGE TIP:** This dish is best if consumed immediately, but leftover fish and vegetables can be stored in separate airtight containers in the refrigerator for up to 3 days.

PER SERVING (3 OUNCES COD + 2 TABLESPOONS DICED RED ONION + ¼ CUP SLICED AVOCADO + ½ CUP CAULIFLOWER RICE): Calories: 177; Protein: 14g; Fat: 11g; Carbohydrates: 7g; Fiber: 5g; Sugar: 3g; Sodium: 414mg

Salmon Cakes and Leafy Greens

SERVES 6 / PREP TIME: 10 MINUTES / COOK TIME: 35 MINUTES

Salmon is full of omega-3 fatty acids that provide antioxidant power to every meal. But maybe you're tired of eating the same old baked or broiled salmon with lemon and pepper. This salmon cake recipe puts a twist on your typical salmon dish and makes it perfect for a portable lunch or dinner meal.

Nonstick cooking spray

2 tablespoons extra-virgin olive oil, divided

½ cup chopped yellow onion

12 ounces canned salmon, drained

1 large egg

1 tablespoon freshly squeezed lemon juice

1 teaspoon garlic powder

1 teaspoon dried parsley

¼ teaspoon salt, plus more for seasoning

1½ cups frozen spinach

Serving Recommendations

SOFT FOODS: about 1 mini salmon cake (about 2 ounces salmon) and ¼ cup spinach

GENERAL: 2 to 3 mini salmon cakes (4 to 6 ounces salmon) and ½ cup spinach, or more as tolerated

1. Preheat the oven at 425°F. Line a baking sheet with parchment paper or aluminum foil and coat with cooking spray.

2. In a medium skillet, heat 1 tablespoon of olive oil over medium heat. Add the onion to the skillet and cook for 5 to 7 minutes or until it is translucent. Remove from heat.

3. Combine the onion, salmon, egg, lemon juice, garlic powder, parsley, and salt. Form into 6 patties.

4. Place the patties on the baking sheet 1 to 2 inches apart and bake for about 25 minutes.

5. While salmon cakes are baking, place the frozen spinach in the same small skillet. Cover and cook for 3 to 4 minutes over medium heat until the spinach softens. Drain the water from the pan. Add the remaining oil and salt to spinach and toss.

6. When the salmon cakes are golden brown, remove them from the oven and serve over spinach.

STORAGE TIP: Store leftover spinach in an airtight container in the refrigerator for up to 7 days and leftover salmon separately in an airtight container in the refrigerator for up to 3 days.

PER SERVING (1 MINI CAKE + ¼ CUP SPINACH): Calories: 160; Protein: 17g; Fat: 9g; Carbohydrates: 3; Fiber: 1g; Sugar: 1g; Sodium: 402mg

Southwest Salmon and Roasted Red Onion and Peppers

SERVES 4 / PREP TIME: 10 MINUTES / COOK TIME: 30 MINUTES

Spice up your salmon with southwest flavor. If you want to enjoy the healthy fats from salmon but are getting bored with your simple salt-and-pepper preparation, add a bit of flavor with fresh onions, peppers, and a variety of herbs and spices. Pair with your favorite steamed veggies if you prefer.

1 medium red bell pepper, sliced in strips

1 medium red onion, cut in ¼-inch slices

2 teaspoons chopped fresh cilantro

2 teaspoons garlic powder

1 teaspoon chili powder

¼ teaspoon salt

Dash freshly ground black pepper *(optional)*

1 pound salmon fillet, cut into 4-ounce pieces

1 tablespoon extra-virgin olive oil

Serving Recommendations
GENERAL: 1 full serving

1. Preheat the oven to 375°F. Line a baking sheet with parchment paper.

2. Place the peppers and onions on the prepared sheet pan and cover with foil. Bake the vegetables for about 15 minutes, but don't turn off the oven when this first timer goes off.

3. While the vegetables are cooking, in a small bowl, mix the cilantro, garlic powder, chili powder, salt, and pepper (if using). Coat the top of each piece of salmon with this mixture.

4. Open the oven when first timer goes off and add salmon pieces skin-side down on the baking sheet. Drizzle fish and veggies with oil.

5. Bake for another 12 to 15 minutes, until the fish flakes easily with a fork. Remove the pan and serve the salmon on top of the vegetables.

STORAGE TIP: Store leftover vegetables in an airtight container in the refrigerator for up to 7 days and the salmon in a separate airtight container in the refrigerator for up to 3 days.

PER SERVING (4 OUNCES SALMON + ½ CUP VEGETABLES):
Calories: 235; Protein: 24g; Fat: 13g; Carbohydrates: 6g; Fiber: 1g; Sugar: 2g; Sodium: 196mg

Maryland-Style Crab Cakes

SERVES 4 / PREP TIME: 6 MINUTES / COOK TIME: 10 MINUTES

You may have had a crab cake before. But you haven't had a crab cake until you've had a Maryland-style crab cake. And I don't mean a cup of mayonnaise, bread crumbs, and parsley. I mean lump crab meat, mustard, just a bit of mayo, and Old Bay seasoning. You don't need a lot of ingredients for a delicious crab cake. Broil with low-carbohydrate veggies like zucchini for a balanced meal you can enjoy any time of day.

Nonstick cooking spray

1 cup zucchini cut in ¼-inch slices

1 tablespoon extra-virgin olive oil

Dash salt

1 cup blue crab meat

2 tablespoons yellow mustard

2 tablespoons light mayonnaise

1 large egg

1 teaspoon Old Bay seasoning

Serving Recommendations

SOFT FOODS: 1 full serving (1 cake and ¼ cup zucchini)

GENERAL: 1 to 2 full servings (1 to 2 cakes and ¼ to ½ cup zucchini)

1. Set an oven rack 6 inches away from the broiler element, then preheat the broiler to high. Line a baking sheet with aluminum foil sprayed with nonstick cooking spray.

2. In a small bowl, toss the zucchini, olive oil, and salt. Arrange on one side of the prepared baking sheet.

3. In another bowl, combine the crab, mustard, mayonnaise, egg, and Old Bay seasoning. Form into 4 evenly sized patties and arrange on the other side of the baking sheet.

4. Broil for about 10 minutes. Crab cakes should be golden brown on top and the zucchini will be tender.

5. Remove from the heat and serve.

STORAGE TIP: Store leftover vegetables in an airtight container in the refrigerator for up to 7 days and the crab cakes in a separate airtight container in the refrigerator for up to 3 days.

PER SERVING (2-OUNCE CRAB CAKE + ¼ CUP ZUCCHINI): Calories: 123; Protein: 14g; Fat: 8g; Carbohydrates: 2g; Fiber: <1g; Sugar: 3g; Sodium: 511mg

Maryland-Style Vegetable Crab Soup

SERVES 8 / PREP TIME: 10 MINUTES / COOK TIME: 1 HOUR+

Maryland-style crab soup is a traditional seafood soup. Those not from the state of Maryland have attempted to imitate it, but it is just not the same as the soup I eat when I visit home. This soup contains the classic Old Bay seasoning that gives everything it touches a delicious savory taste like no other. And remember to use blue crab only in this recipe. Phillips crab meat is recommended. Reduce the amount of sodium in this recipe by adding less seasoning, crab, or salt.

1 tablespoon extra-virgin olive oil

2 cups peeled, sliced carrot

1 cup chopped yellow onion

6 cups reduced-sodium beef or vegetable broth

1 pound claw blue crab meat

1 (15-ounce) can diced tomatoes, drained

3 teaspoons Old Bay seasoning

¼ teaspoon salt

Serving Recommendations
SOFT FOODS: ½ cup to 1 cup
GENERAL: 1 to 2 cups

1. In a medium saucepan, heat the olive oil over medium heat and add carrot and onion. Cook for about 7 minutes, until the onion is translucent. Transfer the veggies to a large pot.

2. Add broth, crab meat, tomato, Old Bay seasoning, and salt. Simmer on low-medium heat for about an hour before serving. Simmer longer, if preferred, to enhance flavor.

INGREDIENT TIP: Add extra low-carbohydrate vegetables like green beans, celery, and cabbage, if this texture is tolerated. Also, if you can tolerate solid meats well, you are welcome to add stewed beef to the recipe, as this is usually what is added in my family's crab soup recipe.

STORAGE TIP: Store leftovers in an airtight container in the refrigerator for up to 3 days.

PER SERVING (1 CUP): Calories: 105; Protein: 13g; Fat: 2g; Carbohydrates: 8g; Fiber: 2g; Sugar: 5g; Sodium: 762mg

Crab Imperial–Topped Roasted Tomatoes

SERVES 4 / PREP TIME: 5 MINUTES / COOK TIME: 20 MINUTES

If you love cheesy mushrooms or stuffed peppers, you'll love this delicious Maryland-style crab imperial over fresh roasted tomatoes. Crab imperial is a decadent and creamy crab recipe, but it is usually full of fat. This take on the crab imperial recipe uses nonfat Greek yogurt instead, so you can enjoy a similar flavor with less fat and calories.

Nonstick cooking spray

2 medium
tomatoes, halved

¼ cup lump blue crab meat

2 tablespoons nonfat plain
Greek yogurt

2 tablespoons almond flour

3 teaspoons light
mayonnaise

1½ tablespoons raw egg

1 tablespoon
coconut aminos

¾ teaspoon freshly
squeezed lemon juice

½ teaspoon Old Bay
seasoning

½ teaspoon yellow mustard
or Dijon mustard

½ teaspoon chopped
fresh parsley

Serving Recommendations
SOFT FOODS: about 1 serving
GENERAL: 1 to 2 servings

1. Preheat the oven to 375°F. Line a baking sheet with aluminum foil and spray with nonstick cooking spray.

2. Scoop out the seeds in each tomato. Arrange the tomato halves on the baking sheet, about an inch or so apart.

3. In a small bowl, combine the crab, yogurt, almond flour, mayonnaise, egg, coconut aminos, lemon juice, Old Bay seasoning, mustard, and parsley. Combine all ingredients well and place a heaping tablespoon of mix in each tomato half. If there is extra mix left, distribute it evenly among the tomatoes.

4. Bake for about 20 minutes. Remove from the oven and enjoy while warm.

SERVING TIP: Feel free to add shredded Cheddar cheese on top of the crab mixture before baking if you prefer.

PER SERVING (1 CRAB-TOPPED TOMATO): Calories: 119; Protein: 12g; Fat: 6g; Carbohydrates: 7; Fiber: 1g; Sugar: 4g; Sodium: 402mg

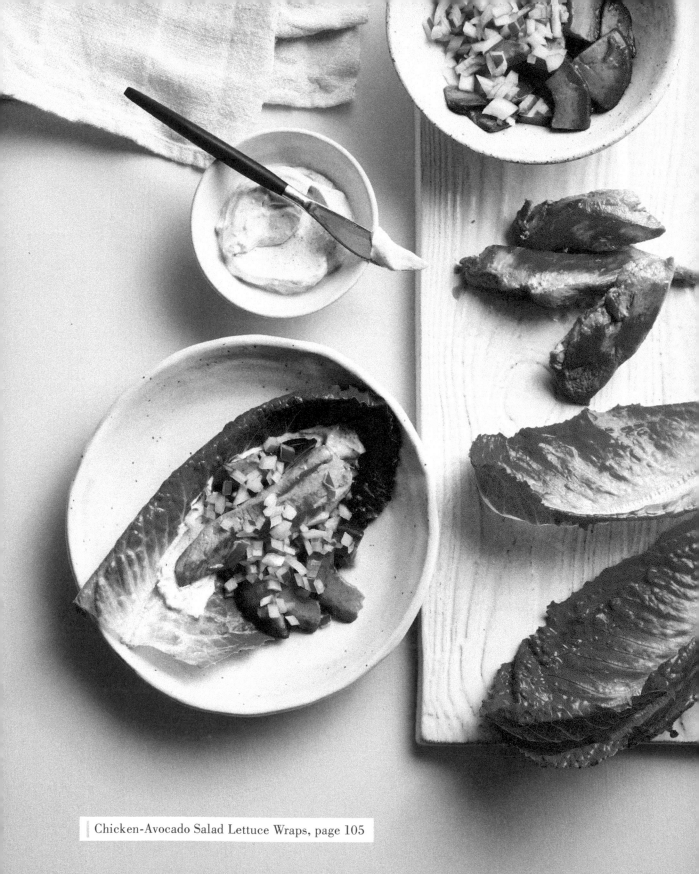

Chicken-Avocado Salad Lettuce Wraps, page 105

Poultry

Almond-Crusted Chicken Tenders

SERVES 4 / PREP TIME: 10 MINUTES / COOK TIME: 35 MINUTES

If you're craving juicy chicken tenders but need to watch your carbohydrate intake, these almond-crusted chicken tenders can fill that void. Not only do you get a juicy chicken tender, but the batter has a nutty flavor. Enjoy with a low-carbohydrate dip such as mustard or Avocado Mayo (page 160) or with a side of roasted butternut squash instead of fries.

Nonstick cooking spray
¾ cup almond
  flour, divided
¼ cup cornstarch
½ teaspoon salt
2 large eggs
16 ounces boneless,
  skinless chicken tenders

Serving Recommendations
GENERAL: 1 full serving

1. Preheat the oven to 400°F. Coat a baking sheet with nonstick cooking spray or parchment paper.

2. While the oven preheats, prepare one plate with ½ cup almond flour, and a second plate with ¼ cup almond flour, cornstarch, and salt. In a small bowl, beat the eggs.

3. With the baking sheet next to your prepping station, coat each side of each chicken tender with the cornstarch and almond flour mixture first, then coat well in egg, and finally coat with the almond flour. Place the battered tender on the baking sheet. Repeat this process for all chicken tenders.

4. Bake for about 35 minutes, turning the tenders over at the halfway point of cooking time, when the batter begins to brown. Serve immediately.

STORAGE TIP: Store leftovers in an airtight container in the refrigerator up to 3 days. When reheating, place in oven at 350°F for 7 to 10 minutes to restore the crispiness of the batter.

PER SERVING (4 OUNCES CHICKEN TENDERS): Calories: 296; Protein: 31g; Fat: 14g; Carbohydrates: 12g; Fiber: 2g; Sugar: 1g; Sodium: 697mg

Cheesy Chicken Meatballs

SERVES 4 / PREP TIME: 10 MINUTES / COOK TIME: 30 MINUTES

These chicken meatballs are tender, juicy, and full of flavor. Their low-carbohydrate profile fits any bariatric post-op stage, while their texture is soft enough for the first few months after surgery. Not to mention that this recipe is simple to prep and fast to cook. To make it a complete meal, serve on top of cooked leafy greens like spinach or kale.

Nonstick cooking spray
1 pound ground chicken
2 tablespoons grated
    Parmesan cheese
2 teaspoons Italian
    seasoning
½ teaspoon garlic powder
1 teaspoon extra-virgin
    olive oil
¼ cup diced yellow onion
2 large eggs

Serving Recommendations
SOFT: 3 meatballs

GENERAL: 3 to 6 meatballs, depending on your daily calorie needs and tolerance

1. Preheat the oven to 400°F. Line a baking sheet with parchment paper or aluminum foil and spray with cooking spray.

2. In a large bowl, combine the ground chicken, Parmesan cheese, Italian seasoning, and garlic powder and mix well. Set aside.

3. In a small skillet, heat the oil over medium-high heat. Cook the onion, stirring frequently, for 5 minutes or until translucent. Remove from heat. Add the cooked onion to the meatball mixture.

4. In a small bowl, beat the eggs. Add to the meatball mixture and combine well.

5. Using a measuring spoon, scoop out 2 tablespoons of the ground chicken mixture and form into a round meatball shape. Repeat this to create 12 meatballs. Place the meatballs on the prepared baking sheet about an inch apart.

6. Cook in the oven for 25 to 30 minutes, until golden brown. Enjoy warm.

> **STORAGE TIP:** Store leftover meatballs in an airtight container and refrigerate for up to 3 days.

PER SERVING (3 MEATBALLS): Calories: 263; Protein: 53g; Fat: 17g; Carbohydrates: 2g; Fiber: <1g; Sugar: 7g; Sodium: 763mg

Harvest Vegetable Chicken Soup

SERVES 8 / PREP TIME: 10 MINUTES / COOK TIME: 3 HOURS

Whether it's a cold winter's day or you're just craving some comfort food, this soup is the perfect option. This simple, yet flavorful soup is easy to make and is a refreshing, low-sodium version of traditional chicken soup. If you don't want to use a whole chicken, substitute with cooked shredded rotisserie chicken.

Nonstick cooking spray

2 cups carrot, peeled and sliced into ½-inch-thick slices

2 cups diced celery

1 cup diced yellow onion

1 (5- to 7-pound) whole chicken

8 cups chicken broth, store-bought or Harvest Vegetable Chicken Bone Broth (page 25)

1¼ teaspoons salt

2 bay leaves

Serving Recommendations

SOFT FOODS: ½ to 1 cup

GENERAL: 1 to 2 cups, or more depending on your daily calorie needs

1. Preheat the oven to 400°F. Coat a roasting pan with nonstick cooking spray.

2. In the roasting pan, arrange the carrot, celery, and onion around the outside. Place the whole chicken in the pan and roast for about 90 minutes or more (about 20 minutes per pound of chicken), until a thermometer inserted in the thigh reads 165°F and the juices run clear.

3. Remove the pan from the oven and remove meat from the carcass, shredding 2 cups of the meat. Reserve the remaining leftover chicken meat for other recipes and the carcass to make Harvest Vegetable Chicken Bone Broth.

4. Transfer the 2 cups chicken and the vegetables to the pot, add the broth, salt, and bay leaves, and bring to a rolling boil over medium high.

5. Simmer over medium heat for at least 1 to 2 hours until the flavors meld. Supervise the pot during the simmering process.

6. Remove the bay leaves and serve.

STORAGE TIP: Store leftovers in a freezer- and microwave-safe container and refrigerate for up to 3 days or freeze for up to 6 months.

PER SERVING (1 CUP): Calories: 90; Protein: 8g; Fat: 3g; Carbohydrates: 7g; Fiber: 2g; Sugar: 4g; Sodium: 231mg

Chicken-Avocado Salad Lettuce Wraps

SERVES 4 / PREP TIME: 10 MINUTES / COOK TIME: 10 MINUTES

A sandwich wrap is a convenient lunchtime meal, but the wrap itself can be high in carbohydrates and calories. Therefore, just replace the wrap with a romaine lettuce leaf and cut the calories dramatically. If you can't tolerate raw vegetables, then feel free to just enjoy the chicken salad and avocado alone.

For the wraps

1 tablespoon extra-virgin olive oil

8 ounces boneless, skinless chicken breast, cut into 2-ounce strips

4 romaine lettuce leaves

4 tablespoons avocado, sliced

½ cup diced red onion

For the spread

4 tablespoons nonfat plain Greek yogurt

½ teaspoon ground cumin

¼ teaspoon salt

Serving Recommendations
GENERAL: 1 to 2 full servings, depending on your daily calorie needs and tolerance

To make the wraps

1. In a medium skillet, heat the oil over medium heat. Cook the chicken strips for about 5 minutes on each side until the chicken is no longer pink. Remove from heat.

2. Place the chicken in the lettuce leaves. Top with avocado and onion.

To make the spread

3. In a small bowl, combine the yogurt, cumin, and salt until fully incorporated. Spread the yogurt mixture over the chicken. Wrap the chicken in the lettuce leaves and enjoy.

STORAGE TIP: Store leftovers in an airtight container in the refrigerator for up to 3 days.

PER SERVING (2 OUNCES CHICKEN + 1 TABLESPOON EACH OF AVOCADO AND SPREAD + 2 TABLESPOONS ONION + 1 LETTUCE LEAF): Calories: 168; Protein: 20g; Fat: 6g; Carbohydrates: 9g; Fiber: 2g; Sugar: <1g; Sodium: 206mg

Chicken Cauliflower Fried Rice

SERVES 8 / PREP TIME: 10 MINUTES / COOK TIME: 45 MINUTES

Fried rice is a takeout favorite but can be full of fat and excess calories. With a few modifications, this classic dish can become a staple meal in your healthy lifestyle. Just replace white rice with cauliflower rice for fewer carbohydrates and more fiber. Then, load the dish with skinless chicken breast for plenty of protein. If you prefer less sodium, use a low-sodium soy sauce.

8 ounces boneless, skinless chicken breast

1 tablespoon extra-virgin olive oil

2 cups cauliflower rice

1 cup peeled, diced carrot

1 cup chopped yellow onion

2 large eggs

8 teaspoons coconut aminos

1 teaspoon garlic powder

1 teaspoon ginger powder

¼ teaspoon salt or 2 teaspoons soy sauce

Serving Recommendations

SOFT FOODS: ½ to 1 full serving (about ½ cup dish)

GENERAL: 1 to 2 full servings, depending on tolerance and daily calorie needs

1. Place the chicken breast in a medium pot. Place water in the pot until it covers the chicken and bring to a boil over medium-high heat. Reduce the heat to medium and cook, covered, for about 30 minutes, until cooked through.

2. Remove the chicken from the heat, drain the water, and rinse with cold water. In a medium bowl, shred the chicken breast and set aside.

3. In a large skillet, heat the olive oil over medium heat. Cook the cauliflower rice, carrot, and onion for 7 to 9 minutes, until softened.

4. Add in the eggs and stir until scrambled in the vegetable mixture for 1 to 2 minutes.

5. Add the shredded chicken, coconut aminos, garlic powder, ginger powder, and salt or soy sauce and cook for another 1 to 2 minutes before serving.

STORAGE TIP: Store leftovers in an airtight container in the refrigerator for up to 3 days.

PER SERVING (⅔ CUP): Calories: 126; Protein: 12g; Fat: 5g; Carbohydrates: 8g; Fiber: 2g; Sugar: 4g; Sodium: 239mg

Sweet Ginger Chicken Stir-Fry

SERVES 4 / PREP TIME: 10 MINUTES / COOK TIME: 20 MINUTES

If you enjoy a sweet sauce on your stir-fry but are trying to limit sugar in your diet, this stir-fry will help fill that void. Instead of using thick, sweet sauces or brown sugar, this recipe uses coconut aminos for flavoring. This coconut sap–derived condiment provides a uniquely and subtly sweet flavor perfect for this recipe.

1 tablespoon extra-virgin
   olive oil
8 ounces skinless boneless
   chicken breast, diced
2 cups peeled,
   chopped carrot
1 cup chopped
   yellow onion
8 teaspoons
   coconut aminos
1 teaspoon garlic powder
1 teaspoon ginger powder
¼ teaspoon salt

Serving Recommendations
GENERAL: 1 to 1½ cups mixture, or more depending on tolerance and daily calorie needs

1. In a large skillet, heat the oil over medium heat. Add the chicken and cook for 5 to 7 minutes, until browned.

2. Add the carrot and onion to the skillet. Cover and cook for another 5 to 7 minutes, or until the onion is slightly translucent and the chicken is cooked through. Stir every 30 seconds or so. (Add a few tablespoons of water to the skillet during cooking if the onion starts to burn or stick to the skillet prior to the carrot softening.)

3. Sprinkle in the coconut aminos, garlic powder, ginger powder, and salt. Add in a few tablespoons of water. Stir the mixture and replace lid for another 2 to 3 minutes. Remove from heat and serve over cauliflower rice or your favorite low-carbohydrate vegetable.

STORAGE TIP: Store leftovers in an airtight container in the refrigerator for up to 3 days.

PER SERVING (½ CUP): Calories: 166; Protein: 19g; Fat: 5g; Carbohydrates: 13g; Fiber: 3g; Sugar: 7g; Sodium: 422mg

Lemon-Pepper Chicken Bake

SERVES 4 / PREP TIME: 10 MINUTES / COOK TIME: 1 HOUR

This one-pan meal makes dinner prep less stressful and more delicious. Its unique flavor of savory and tart make it a chicken dish unlike any other you've had before. Seasonings are kept simple to allow the natural flavor of the vegetables to shine through. To save time, you can prep this pan meal ahead of time and store it in the refrigerator covered with plastic wrap for 24 hours. For more volume and fiber, add other low-carbohydrate vegetables such as bell pepper, butternut squash, or carrot.

8 ounces skinless chicken breast tenders
1 cup sliced zucchini
1 medium tomato, quartered
1 medium red onion, quartered
1 lemon, sliced
1 tablespoon extra-virgin olive oil
1 teaspoon seasoned salt
Freshly ground black pepper

Serving Recommendations
GENERAL: 1 full serving

1. Preheat the oven to 400°F.

2. In a casserole dish, place the chicken breasts and arrange the zucchini, tomato, onion, and lemon slices around the breasts. Drizzle the entire dish with olive oil. Toss all the ingredients to make sure they are lightly coated with oil.

3. Sprinkle seasoned salt and pepper over the entire dish.

4. Bake for about 1 hour, until the vegetables are softened and slightly charred and the chicken is cooked through. (It should show an internal temperature of 165°F and the juices run clear.)

5. Remove from the oven and enjoy.

> **STORAGE TIP:** Store leftovers together in an airtight container in the refrigerator for up to 3 days.

PER SERVING (2 OUNCES CHICKEN + ¾ CUP VEGETABLES):
Calories: 131; Protein: 17g; Fat: 5g; Carbohydrates: 6g; Fiber: 1g; Sugar: 4g; Sodium: 440mg

Chicken and Zucchini Noodle "Alfredo"

SERVES 5 / PREP TIME: 10 MINUTES / COOK TIME: 15 MINUTES

Comfort food may be missing from most healthy lifestyle plans, but it doesn't have to be. By using Vegan Garlic Cream Sauce (page 162) instead of your traditional alfredo sauce, you reduce fat and calories without sacrificing flavor. By using zucchini noodles instead of linguine or fettucine, you cut carbohydrates dramatically while adding extra fiber to this tasty dish.

1 tablespoon extra-virgin olive oil

8 ounces ground chicken

1 recipe Vegan Garlic Cream Sauce (page 162)

1 teaspoon garlic powder

¼ teaspoon salt

Nonstick cooking spray

2 medium zucchini, peeled and spiralized

Serving Recommendations
GENERAL: 1 full serving, or more depending on your daily calorie needs and tolerance

1. In a medium skillet, heat the oil over medium heat. Add the ground chicken and cook for 7 to 9 minutes, until the chicken is no longer pink.

2. Add the Vegan Garlic Cream Sauce to the skillet and toss with the chicken. Add in garlic powder and salt. Transfer to a medium bowl and set aside.

3. Wipe the skillet of any residual sauce and spray the same skillet with nonstick cooking spray. Place the zucchini into the skillet and cook, stirring frequently, for 4 to 5 minutes, until softened a bit. Remove from the heat and set aside on a serving plate.

4. Serve the sauce over the top of the zucchini noodles.

STORAGE TIP: Store leftover zucchini noodles and sauce in separate airtight containers in the refrigerator for up to 3 days.

PER SERVING (½ CUP ZUCCHINI NOODLES + ¼ CUP GROUND CHICKEN + ¼ CUP SAUCE): Calories: 156; Protein: 17g; Fat: 8g; Carbohydrates: 6g; Fiber: 2g; Sugar: 2g; Sodium: 340mg

Chicken Parmesan with Diced Tomatoes

SERVES 4 / PREP TIME: 10 MINUTES / COOK TIME: 25 MINUTES

Chicken Parmesan is a classic Italian dish usually served over a large bed of pasta. But if you're cutting carbohydrates, you may feel like you won't be able to enjoy this dish again. However, by using almond flour for breading, baking the chicken instead of frying, and serving with veggies instead of pasta, you can have the flavor of this dish in a healthy, protein-packed form.

Nonstick cooking spray

1 tablespoon cornstarch

½ teaspoon salt, divided

4 tablespoons almond flour

1 teaspoon garlic powder

½ teaspoon Italian seasoning, divided

1 large egg

8 ounces boneless, skinless chicken breast, cut into 2-ounce tenders

2 tablespoons extra-virgin olive oil, divided

½ cup shredded Parmesan cheese

1 cup sliced zucchini

1 cup chopped tomatoes

Serving Recommendations
GENERAL: 1 to 2 full servings, depending on tolerance and daily calorie needs

1. Preheat the oven to 400°F. Coat a baking sheet with cooking spray or line with parchment paper and set aside.

2. Prepare one plate with cornstarch and ¼ teaspoon salt, and another plate with almond flour, garlic powder, and ¼ teaspoon Italian seasoning combined. Beat the egg well in a small bowl and set it between the plates.

3. Coat each side of each chicken tender with cornstarch first, then coat well in egg, and finally coat with the almond flour mixture. Place the battered tender on the sheet. Repeat this process for all chicken tenders.

4. Using a basting brush, brush the tenders on both sides with 1 tablespoon olive oil. Sprinkle the tenders with Parmesan cheese. Bake for 20 to 25 minutes, or until golden brown.

5. While chicken tenders are cooking, in a medium skillet, heat the remaining 1 tablespoon oil over medium heat. Add the zucchini and sprinkle with remaining ¼ teaspoon salt. Cook for about 5 minutes, stirring frequently, until the zucchini starts to soften.

6. Add the tomatoes and remaining ¼ teaspoon Italian seasoning and cook for another 3 to 4 minutes, stirring frequently.

7. Remove the chicken from the heat and serve by pouring a portion of the zucchini and tomato mixture over the chicken.

> **STORAGE TIP:** Store leftovers in an airtight container in the refrigerator up to 3 days. When reheating, place in oven at 350°F for 7 to 10 minutes to restore the crispiness of the chicken.

PER SERVING (2 TENDERS + ½ CUP ZUCCHINI AND TOMATOES):
Calories: 250; Protein: 25g; Fat: 13g; Carbohydrates: 10g; Fiber: 2g; Sugar: 3g; Sodium: 552mg

Turkey and Strawberry-Spinach Salad

SERVES 4 / PREP TIME: 5 MINUTES / COOK TIME: 10 MINUTES

Once you're able to tolerate raw vegetables, this simple salad recipe will give you a fresh take on your typical garden-variety salad meal. Tossing savory turkey with fresh and sweet strawberries makes for a delicious combination, especially when drizzled with the rich, but refreshing flavor of balsamic vinaigrette.

1 tablespoon extra-virgin olive oil

8 ounces boneless, skinless turkey breast tenderloin, cut into 1-ounce strips

2 cups baby spinach leaves

1 cup sliced strawberries (8 large strawberries)

¼ cup balsamic vinaigrette

¼ cup goat cheese crumbles

Dash freshly ground black pepper

Serving Recommendations
GENERAL: 1 to 2 full servings, depending on your daily calorie needs and tolerance

1. In a medium skillet, heat the oil over medium heat. Cook the turkey for about 3 minutes on each side until the turkey is cooked through. Remove from the heat.

2. Place the spinach in a large serving bowl. Place the strawberry slices and turkey on top and drizzle with the balsamic vinaigrette. Top with the goat cheese and pepper, then serve.

STORAGE TIP: If you plan on having leftovers, then prep the ingredients and store them separately in airtight containers in the refrigerator, so the baby spinach leaves don't get soggy from sitting in the vinaigrette. Store for up to 3 days.

PER SERVING (2 OUNCES TURKEY + ½ CUP BABY SPINACH LEAVES + ¼ CUP STRAWBERRY SLICES + 1 TABLESPOON EACH OF GOAT CHEESE CRUMBLES AND VINAIGRETTE): Calories: 176; Protein: 18g; Fat: 9g; Carbohydrates: 5g; Fiber: 1g; Sugar: 3g; Sodium: 133mg

Turkey Lettuce Wrap

SERVES 4 / PREP TIME: 10 MINUTES / COOK TIME: 10 MINUTES

A turkey sandwich is a go-to quick-and-healthy lunch option. Fortunately, you can still enjoy this lunchtime classic without bread and without sacrificing the flavor. Instead of bread, enjoy a fiber-filled lettuce wrap; and, instead of mayonnaise, use a flavorful Greek yogurt Caesar dressing. If you want to cut back on fat, simply add less dressing.

1 tablespoon extra-virgin olive oil

8 ounces boneless, skinless turkey breast tenderloin, cut into 2-ounce strips

4 romaine lettuce leaves

2 ounces Swiss cheese (2 slices)

8 thin tomato slices

1 recipe Greek Yogurt Caesar Dressing (page 163)

Serving Recommendations
GENERAL: 1 to 2 full servings, depending on your daily calorie needs and tolerance

1. In a medium skillet, heat the oil over medium heat. Cook the turkey for about 5 minutes on each side until the turkey is cooked through. Remove from the heat.

2. Place a turkey strip into the center of each lettuce leaf. Top each with a ½ slice of Swiss cheese and 2 thin tomato slices. Drizzle each with 2 tablespoons of the dressing.

3. Wrap well and enjoy.

SERVING TIP: If you can't tolerate raw veggies like lettuce, enjoy this turkey dish alone with dressing and cheese.

STORAGE TIP: You should store all ingredients separately in airtight containers in the refrigerator. Consume the turkey within 3 days, tomatoes and lettuce within 7 days, and dressing within 7 days.

PER SERVING (2 OUNCES TURKEY + 2 SLICES TOMATO + ½ OUNCE SWISS CHEESE + 2 TABLESPOONS DRESSING): Calories: 260; Protein: 25g; Fat: 15g; Carbohydrates: 5g; Fiber: 1g; Sugar: 2g; Sodium: 439mg

Crustless Turkey Pot Pie

SERVES 5 / PREP TIME: 10 MINUTES / COOK TIME: 20 MINUTES

Whether it's a cold winter day or just the end of a long and busy week, comfort food warms the soul. Unfortunately, a lot of comfort foods are high in calories, carbohydrates, and fat. That's where this crustless pot pie comes in to save the day. The rich, flavorful gravy complements low-fat turkey and fiber-rich carrot and onion to give you a stick-to-your-ribs meal without the excess calories.

1 tablespoon
   unsalted butter
2 cups peeled, sliced carrot
1 cup diced yellow onion
2 cups chicken broth,
   store-bought or Harvest
   Vegetable Chicken Bone
   Broth (page 25)
¼ cup cornstarch
   mixed with 4 to
   6 tablespoons water
1 pound lean ground turkey
¼ teaspoon garlic powder
¼ teaspoon ground sage
½ teaspoon salt

Serving Recommendations
GENERAL: 1 full serving

1. In a large skillet, heat the butter over medium heat. Add the carrot and onion and cook for 8 minutes, stirring frequently, until the onion becomes translucent.

2. Add the broth and cornstarch slurry. Cook for 2 to 3 minutes, stirring frequently, until the gravy thickens. Set aside.

3. In another large skillet, brown the ground turkey for 8 to 10 minutes over medium heat. Drain the liquid.

4. Add the turkey to the gravy and vegetable mixture and combine well.

5. Add the garlic powder, ground sage, and salt to taste. Stir well and enjoy.

STORAGE TIP: Store in an airtight container in the refrigerator for up to 3 days or freeze for up to 3 months.

PER SERVING (1 CUP): Calories: 243; Protein: 22g; Fat: 9g; Carbohydrates: 19g; Fiber: 4g; Sugar: 6g; Sodium: 400mg

Turkey-Vegetable Burger

SERVES 4 / PREP TIME: 10 MINUTES / COOK TIME: 20 MINUTES

You may have had a turkey burger before, but not like this one. This version is a balanced meal in one patty, with plenty of diced and shredded veggies rolled into a flavorful ground turkey burger. Enjoy alone or with a healthy sauce like Low-Carb Honey Mustard Yogurt Dressing (page 169) for a delicious meal. If you prefer, and if you can tolerate it, feel free to enjoy your burger in a lettuce leaf wrap or low-carbohydrate wrap of your choice.

1 tablespoon extra-virgin olive oil

¼ cup diced bell pepper

¼ cup diced yellow onion

¼ cup shredded carrot

8 ounces lean ground turkey

1 large egg

1 teaspoon garlic powder

1 teaspoon ground cumin

¼ teaspoon salt

Nonstick cooking spray

Serving Recommendations
SOFT FOODS: ½ to 1 burger
GENERAL: 1 to 2 burgers, depending on your daily calorie needs

1. In a medium skillet, heat the oil over medium heat. Cook the bell pepper, onion, and carrot for 5 to 7 minutes or until the onion is slightly translucent. Remove from heat.

2. In a large bowl, combine the ground turkey, egg, garlic powder, cumin, salt, and cooked vegetables. Form the turkey mixture into 4 patties.

3. Place the same skillet over medium heat and spray with nonstick cooking spray.

4. Cook the patties for 4 to 6 minutes on each side or until golden brown. Serve warm.

STORAGE TIP: Store leftovers in an airtight container in the refrigerator for up to 3 days.

PER SERVING (1 BURGER OR 2½ OUNCES): Calories: 142; Protein: 12g; Fat: 9g; Carbohydrates: 2g; Fiber: 1g; Sugar: 1g; Sodium: 203mg

Sage-Spiced Turkey and Cauliflower Rice

SERVES 4 / PREP TIME: 10 MINUTES / COOK TIME: 15 MINUTES

Ground turkey can become boring at mealtime without a dash of flavor. If you're not sure what to use to spice up this healthy protein option, use this recipe which adds ground sage, garlic powder, salt, and chopped sweet yellow onion to give your ground turkey a boost.

1 tablespoon extra-virgin olive oil

1 cup peeled, chopped carrot

½ cup chopped sweet yellow onion

8 ounces lean ground turkey

1 cup cauliflower rice

1 teaspoon garlic powder

½ teaspoon ground sage

¼ teaspoon salt

½ cup water

1. In a medium skillet, heat the oil over medium heat. Cook the carrot and onion for 5 to 7 minutes, or until the onion is slightly translucent.

2. Add the ground turkey, cauliflower rice, garlic powder, sage, and salt to the skillet. Add in the water, and stir veggies and turkey occasionally until the water is absorbed and the cauliflower rice is cooked well, about 7 minutes. Add several table-spoons of water to the skillet during cooking if the mixture starts to stick to the pan before it is finished cooking.

3. Enjoy warm.

Serving Recommendations

SOFT FOODS: ½ cup to 1 cup

GENERAL: 1 to 2 cups

STORAGE TIP: Store leftovers in an airtight container in the refrigerator for up to 3 days.

PER SERVING (¾ CUP): Calories: 144; Protein: 12g; Fat: 8g; Carbohydrates: 6g; Fiber: 2g; Sugar: 3g; Sodium: 216mg

Roasted Turkey Breast and Root Vegetables

SERVES 4 / PREP TIME: 10 MINUTES / COOK TIME: 1 HOUR 30 MINUTES

If you like Thanksgiving dinner but don't want to cook for hours or clean up all the dirty dishes, this one-pan turkey meal is for you. Just a bit of peeling and prepping veggies, a sprinkle of salt, and less than an hour of cooking gives you that holiday dinner taste without the extra work.

Nonstick cooking spray

2 cups baby carrots

1 cup peeled, cubed
   sweet potato

1 cup chopped
   yellow onion

1 tablespoon extra-virgin
   olive oil

¼ teaspoon salt

8 ounces boneless, skinless
   turkey breast

Serving Recommendations
GENERAL: 1 to 2 full servings, depending on your daily calorie needs and tolerance

1. Preheat the oven to 350°F. Line a medium to large shallow roasting pan with aluminum foil and coat with nonstick cooking spray.

2. In a medium mixing bowl, toss the carrots, sweet potatoes, and onion in the oil. Sprinkle with the salt, coating all vegetables well.

3. Arrange the turkey breast and vegetables in the pan and cook for 60 to 90 minutes, or until the internal temperature of the turkey breast is 165°F.

4. Slice the turkey breast before serving and measure out your veggies. Enjoy.

STORAGE TIP: Store the leftovers in an airtight container in the refrigerator for up to 3 days.

PER SERVING (2 OUNCES TURKEY BREAST + ½ TO ¾ CUP VEGGIES):
Calories: 164; Protein: 18g; Fat: 5g; Carbohydrates: 11g; Fiber: 3g; Sugar: 3g; Sodium: 259mg

Savory Turkey and Carrot "Linguine"

SERVES 5 / PREP TIME: 10 MINUTES / COOK TIME: 15 MINUTES

If you're craving noodles and are trying to limit carbohydrates in your diet, but you're tired of zucchini noodles, try this carrot "linguine" recipe. With simple ingredients like onion and turkey tossed in Vegan Garlic Cream Sauce (page 162), this dish provides the taste of a creamy pasta with plenty of protein and fiber and fewer carbohydrates.

1 tablespoon extra-virgin olive oil, divided

10 ounces lean ground turkey

⅔ cup peeled, chopped yellow onion

¼ teaspoon salt, divided

5 medium (about 6-inch long) carrots, peeled

1 recipe Vegan Garlic Cream Sauce (page 162)

Serving Recommendations
GENERAL: 1 to 2 full servings, depending on your daily calorie needs and tolerance

1. In a medium skillet, heat 1½ teaspoons of oil over medium. Cook the turkey and onion for 7 to 9 minutes, or until the onion is slightly translucent and the turkey is cooked. Sprinkle in ⅛ teaspoon of the salt and mix well. Remove and set aside.

2. Using a vegetable peeler or spiralizer, cut the carrots into long, thin, flat noodles.

3. In the same skillet, heat the remaining oil and add in the carrot "linguine." Cook until slightly softened, 3 to 4 minutes, stirring frequently. Place the carrots on serving plate or in a bowl.

4. In the same skillet, warm the garlic sauce for 2 to 3 minutes on low-to-medium heat, stirring frequently. Add the ground turkey, onion, and remaining ⅛ teaspoon salt to the saucepan. Combine well.

5. Serve the sauce over the carrot "linguine."

STORAGE TIP: Store in an airtight container in the refrigerator for up to 5 days.

PER SERVING (½ CUP CARROT "LINGUINE" + ¼ CUP GROUND TURKEY AND ONION MIXTURE + ¼ CUP SAUCE): Calories: 183; Protein: 16g; Fat: 9g; Carbohydrates: 12g; Fiber: 3g; Sugar: 3g; Sodium: 323mg

Zucchini Noodles and Turkey Marinara

SERVES 4 / PREP TIME: 10 MINUTES / COOK TIME: 20 MINUTES

Pasta is typically not tolerated well after bariatric surgery. Zucchini noodles provide a low-carbohydrate alternative, while adding antioxidants and fiber that processed pasta would not provide. If you don't have a spiralizer, you can use a vegetable peeler to make flat strips of zucchini for use as a noodle alternative.

1 tablespoon extra-virgin olive oil

8 ounces boneless, skinless turkey breast tenderloin, diced

1 cup diced yellow onion

¼ teaspoon salt, plus more for seasoning

2 medium zucchini, peeled and spiralized

1 cup canned diced tomatoes, drained

1 teaspoon garlic powder

½ teaspoon Italian seasoning

½ cup shredded mozzarella cheese

Serving Recommendations
GENERAL: 1 to 2 full servings, depending on your daily calorie needs and tolerance

1. In a medium skillet, heat the oil over medium heat. Cook the turkey and onion for 7 to 9 minutes, or until the onion is slightly translucent and the turkey is cooked. Sprinkle with the salt and combine well. Remove the mixture and set aside.

2. In the same skillet, place the zucchini and cook, stirring frequently, for 4 to 5 minutes, or until zucchini is softened. Remove from the heat and set the noodles aside on a serving plate.

3. Add the tomato, garlic powder, and Italian seasoning to a blender and blend on low for 15 to 20 seconds. Pour into the same skillet and heat on low to warm. Season with salt and stir well. Add in the turkey and onion mixture and warm for another 2 to 3 minutes.

4. Remove from heat, pour over zucchini noodles, top with mozzarella cheese, and serve.

> **STORAGE TIP:** Store the sauce and zucchini in separate airtight containers in the refrigerator for up to 3 days.

PER SERVING (⅔ CUP SAUCE + ½ CUP ZUCCHINI NOODLES + 1 TABLESPOON CHEESE): Calories: 191; Protein: 21g; Fat: 8g; Carbohydrates: 8g; Fiber: 2g; Sugar: 5g; Sodium: 697mg

Brown Sugar and Citrus Baked Pork Chops
with Roasted Vegetables, page 126

CHAPTER SEVEN

Pork and Beef

Ground Pork with Goat Cheese and Spinach

SERVES 4 / PREP TIME: 5 MINUTES / COOK TIME: 15 MINUTES

Add an upscale twist to your typical ground pork recipes with creamy goat cheese and spinach. This combination, along with a simple blend of spices, provides satisfying flavor with plenty of protein and a dash of antioxidants from the leafy greens. Add more spinach or other low-carbohydrate vegetables, like chopped bell pepper or broccoli, if desired.

1 tablespoon extra-virgin olive oil

8 ounces lean ground pork

2 cups frozen spinach

4 ounces crumbled goat cheese

1 teaspoon garlic powder

¼ teaspoon salt

Serving Recommendations

SOFT FOODS: ½ cup to 1 cup

GENERAL: about 1 cup, or more depending on daily calorie needs

1. In a large skillet, heat the oil over medium heat. Cook the pork for 7 to 9 minutes, stirring frequently, until cooked through.

2. Add the frozen spinach and cook for 2 to 3 minutes, stirring frequently. Remove the skillet from the heat and drain the fat from the pork.

3. Return the skillet to the heat and add the goat cheese, garlic powder, and salt, stirring frequently until the cheese melts, about 2 minutes. Remove from the heat and enjoy.

STORAGE TIP: Store the leftovers in an airtight container in the refrigerator for up to 3 days.

PER SERVING (½ CUP): Calories: 232; Protein: 18g; Fat: 15g; Carbohydrates: 5g; Fiber: 2g; Sugar: 0g; Sodium: 379mg

Garlic-and-Ginger Pork Stir-Fry

SERVES 4 / PREP TIME: 5 MINUTES / COOK TIME: 15 MINUTES

This simple stir-fry combines pork, green beans, and onion with the unique taste of coconut aminos, which adds flavor without the excess sugar or fat of other stir-fry sauces. Coconut aminos is made from the fermented sap of coconut palm and is usually combined with sea salt to create a lower-sodium savory condiment. This stir-fry option is a good alternative to the beef stir-fry recipe if you're not tolerating solid meats well. Feel free to add more low-carbohydrate vegetables of your choice if you prefer more volume in your stir-fry dish.

1 tablespoon extra-virgin olive oil

1 cup chopped green beans, frozen or fresh

½ cup chopped yellow onion

8 ounces lean ground pork

8 teaspoons coconut aminos

1 teaspoon garlic powder

1 teaspoon ground ginger

¼ teaspoon salt or 2 teaspoons soy sauce

Serving Recommendations
GENERAL: about 1 cup, or more depending on daily calorie needs

1. In a large skillet, heat the oil over medium heat. Cook the green beans, pork, and onion for 7 to 9 minutes, stirring frequently. Remove the skillet from the heat and drain the fat from the pork.

2. Return the skillet to the heat and add the coconut aminos, garlic powder, ground ginger, and salt. Cook for 1 to 2 minutes, stirring frequently, until the vegetables and pork are coated well with the seasoning mixture.

3. Remove from heat and enjoy.

STORAGE TIP: Store in an airtight container in the refrigerator for up to 3 days.

PER SERVING (A LITTLE LESS THAN ½ CUP): Calories: 162; Protein: 12g; Fat: 9g; Carbohydrates: 6g; Fiber: 1g; Sugar: 4g; Sodium: 357mg

Sloppy Joe–Style Ground Pork

SERVES 4 / PREP TIME: 5 MINUTES / COOK TIME: 10 MINUTES

If you like Sloppy Joe sandwiches but are trying to cut down on sugar and carbohydrates, you'll love this low-carbohydrate Sloppy Joe recipe. Just a dash of sweetness from the brown sugar plus the use of lean pork instead of beef will provide the flavor of this lunchtime classic without the extra sugar and calories. Enjoy alone or served over a steamed portion of your favorite low-carbohydrate vegetables, in a lettuce wrap, or over a Savory Cheese Biscuit (page 144).

1 tablespoon extra-virgin olive oil

8 ounces lean ground pork

1 cup chopped yellow onion

1 cup canned diced tomatoes, drained

1 tablespoon apple cider vinegar

1 tablespoon brown sugar

1 teaspoon salt

Serving Recommendations

PUREE: ¼ cup to ½ cup (blend first before enjoying on this texture phase)

SOFT FOODS: ½ cup to 1 cup

GENERAL: about 1 cup, or more depending on daily calorie needs

1. In a large skillet, heat the oil over medium heat. Cook the pork and onion for 7 to 9 minutes, stirring frequently, until cooked through. Remove the skillet from the heat and drain the fat from the pork.

2. Return the skillet to the heat and add the tomatoes, apple cider vinegar, brown sugar, and salt. Reduce the heat to medium low and simmer for 2 minutes. Serve and enjoy.

STORAGE TIP: Store leftovers in an airtight container in the refrigerator for up to 3 days or freeze for up to 3 months.

PER SERVING (½ CUP): Calories: 172; Protein: 13g; Fat: 9g; Carbohydrates: 10g; Fiber: 2g; Sugar: 6g; Sodium: 287mg

Peanut Sauce–Smothered Pork Chops with Roasted Broccoli

SERVES 4 / PREP TIME: 5 MINUTES / COOK TIME: 25 MINUTES

This recipe gives your basic pork chop some Thai-inspired flavor with peanut sauce poured over boneless baked pork chops and paired with a healthy steamed side of broccoli. Feel free to slice the pork chops in strips before serving to make sure the sauce hits every square inch.

Nonstick cooking spray

1 tablespoon extra-virgin olive oil

1 pound boneless pork chops (4 small boneless chops)

2 cups chopped broccoli florets

1 recipe Creamy Peanut Sauce (page 164)

Serving Recommendations
GENERAL: about 1 full serving

1. Preheat the oven to 400°F. Spray a casserole dish or deep pan with nonstick cooking spray and set aside.

2. In a large skillet, heat the oil over medium-high heat. Sear the pork chops for about 3 minutes on each side.

3. Place the seared pork chops and chopped broccoli florets in the casserole dish and bake for 15 to 20 minutes or until the internal temperature of the pork is 145°F and the juices run clear.

4. When the pork is nearly done cooking, use a small saucepan to heat the sauce for 4 to 5 minutes over low heat. Pour over the pork before serving.

STORAGE TIP: Store the pork chops in an airtight container and refrigerate for up to 3 days. Store the sauce in a separate airtight container in the refrigerator for up to 7 days. To reheat the pork, heat at 350°F for 7 to 10 minutes in a shallow pan with a bit of water in the bottom.

PER SERVING (4-OUNCE BONELESS PORK CHOP + ½ CUP BROCCOLI + 3 TABLESPOONS PEANUT SAUCE): Calories: 277; Protein: 28g; Fat: 16g; Carbohydrates: 9g; Fiber: 3g; Sugar: 3g; Sodium: 457mg

Brown Sugar and Citrus Baked Pork Chops with Roasted Vegetables

SERVES 4 / PREP TIME: 5 MINUTES, PLUS 30 MINUTES TO MARINATE / COOK TIME: 25 MINUTES

If you like the combination of sweet and sour, this tart and sweet pork chop recipe will hit the spot. The citrus marinade and thin brown sugar rub used with these pork chops bring a unique flavor profile to an otherwise everyday meat dish. Pair with steamed vegetables or salad to allow a lighter, fiber-rich side to balance out the rich protein content and full flavor of this pork dish.

1 pound boneless pork chops (4 small boneless chops)

Juice of 1 large lemon

2 tablespoons apple cider vinegar

Nonstick cooking spray

1 tablespoon extra-virgin olive oil

8 teaspoons brown sugar

1 teaspoon garlic powder

¼ teaspoon salt

1 cup chopped tomato

1 cup sweet bell pepper, sliced into strips

Serving Recommendations
GENERAL: about 1 full serving

1. Place the pork chops in a shallow dish or sealable 1-gallon storage bag. Cover the pork chops with the lemon juice and apple cider vinegar and cover the shallow dish or seal the bag tightly. Place in the refrigerator for about 30 minutes.

2. Preheat the oven to 400°F. Spray a casserole dish or deep pan with nonstick cooking spray and set aside.

3. In a large skillet, heat the oil over medium-high heat. Sear the pork chops, about 3 minutes on each side, until slightly browned.

4. While the pork sears, in a small bowl, mix the brown sugar, garlic powder, and salt. Spread the brown sugar mixture over one side of the pork chops, then place the pork chops in the casserole dish rubbed-side down.

5. Spread the remaining brown sugar mixture over the top of the pork chops. Arrange the tomato and pepper around the pork chops.

6. Bake the pork chops and vegetables for 15 to 20 minutes or until the internal temperature is 145°F and juices run clear. Serve the pork chops with a side of the tomato and bell pepper.

STORAGE TIP: Store leftovers in an airtight container in the refrigerator for up to 3 days or freeze for up to 3 months. To reheat the pork, preheat the oven to 350°F and heat for 7 to 10 minutes in a shallow pan with a bit of water in the bottom so the pork doesn't dry out.

PER SERVING (4-OUNCE BONELESS PORK CHOP + ½ CUP VEGGIES):
Calories: 224; Protein: 22g; Fat: 10g; Carbohydrates: 14g; Fiber: 1g; Sugar: 11g; Sodium: 292mg

Coconut-Crusted Pork Tenders and Parsnip "Fries"

SERVES 6 / PREP TIME: 10 MINUTES / COOK TIME: 40 MINUTES

You may be used to eating pork tenderloin in little coin-shaped slices with a sauce of some sort. But if you're getting bored with the usual presentation, you'll love this pork tenders recipe, which makes pork tenderloin a more casual option you can enjoy for lunch or dinner. Parsnips make delicious "fries," but if you prefer a lower-carbohydrate option, use baby carrots instead.

For the "fries"

2 cups chopped parsnip (3 parsnips)

1 tablespoon extra-virgin olive oil

¼ teaspoon salt

For the pork

4 tablespoons coconut flour

½ teaspoon ginger powder

¼ teaspoon salt

1 tablespoon cornstarch

1 large egg

12 ounces pork tenderloin, cut into 6 strips

1 tablespoon extra-virgin olive oil

Serving Recommendations
GENERAL: 1 full serving

To make the "fries"

1. Preheat the oven to 400°F. Line a baking sheet with parchment paper and set aside.

2. Place the parsnips in a medium mixing bowl. Add the oil and salt and toss to coat. Spread the parsnips evenly across the baking sheet.

3. Bake for 20 minutes, or until slightly golden brown.

To make the pork

4. While the parsnips bake, on a medium plate, combine the coconut flour, ginger powder, and salt. On a second plate, spread the cornstarch evenly. In a small bowl, beat an egg, and place it in the middle of the two plates.

5. Remove the parsnips from the oven about 20 minutes into cooking and push to one side of the baking sheet.

6. Coat a strip of pork lightly with cornstarch, then coat in beaten egg, and then coat well in the coconut flour mixture. Place on the baking sheet. Repeat until all the pork strips are coated and arranged on the baking sheet. Lightly brush the pork strips with the oil.

7. Bake for about 20 minutes or until the pork tenders are golden brown on top. Remove the baking sheet from the oven and serve the pork tenders with a side of parsnip fries.

STORAGE TIP: Store leftover pork and parsnips in separate airtight containers and refrigerate for up to 3 days or freeze for up to 3 months. To reheat the pork, place in a 350°F oven for about 10 minutes.

PER SERVING (2-OUNCE PORK TENDER + ¼ CUP PARSNIPS):
Calories: 177; Protein: 14g; Fat: 7g; Carbohydrates: 14g; Fiber: 4g; Sugar: 1g; Sodium: 251mg

Sweet Pulled Pork Tenderloin with Shredded Carrots

SERVES 4 / PREP TIME: 10 MINUTES / COOK TIME: 2 HOURS

I associate barbeque with the memories of warm summer days and delicious cookouts. This sweet pulled pork tenderloin dish brings the iconic flavors of summertime into your kitchen any time of the year. Paired with shredded carrot, this dish contains plenty of protein and flavor. While this dish is mostly hands-off until the last half hour, be sure to supervise the pot during the two-hour cook time, adding in water as needed (if any has evaporated during the cooking period) to ensure the pork does not burn.

1 pound pork tenderloin

1 cup shredded carrot

1 tablespoon extra-virgin olive oil

½ cup chopped yellow onion

1 cup canned diced tomatoes, drained

¼ cup brown sugar

2 tablespoons apple cider vinegar

¼ teaspoon salt

Serving Recommendations

SOFT FOODS: ½ to 1 serving (½ to 1 cup meat and 2 to 4 tablespoons sauce)

GENERAL: 1 to 2 full servings, depending on daily calorie needs

1. In a large pot, place the pork tenderloin and cover with water. Cover and simmer over medium-high heat for about 2 hours, or until pork is easily shredded as you stir the pork.

2. About 30 minutes before the 2-hour timer goes off for the pork, add the shredded carrot to the pot.

3. When the pork is about 15 minutes from being done, in a large skillet over medium heat, heat the oil and cook the onion for 5 to 7 minutes, stirring frequently, until translucent.

4. Add in the diced tomatoes, brown sugar, apple cider vinegar, and salt. Simmer for 5 to 7 minutes, until the flavors develop.

5. Remove the onion and tomato mixture from the heat and pour into a blender. Blend on low for 1 to 2 minutes until smooth.

6. Once the pork is cooked, drain any excess water, reduce the heat to low, and add the sauce to the pot. Incorporate the pork with the sauce and simmer for 5 to 10 minutes. Serve warm alone or on a Savory Cheese Biscuit (page 144).

STORAGE TIP: Store leftovers in an airtight container in the refrigerator for up to 3 days.

PER SERVING (1 CUP PULLED PORK AND CARROTS + ¼ CUP SAUCE):
Calories: 209; Protein: 24g; Fat: 6g; Carbohydrates: 15g; Fiber: 1g; Sugar: 13g; Sodium: 294mg

Beef and Swiss Cheesesteak-Style Lettuce Roll-Up

SERVES 4 / PREP TIME: 5 MINUTES / COOK TIME: 10 MINUTES

This lettuce roll-up recipe allows you to enjoy the delicious taste of a cheesesteak sandwich while staying on track with your low-carbohydrate regimen. The bread is replaced with a crisp lettuce wrap, and lean beef and low-sodium cheese are used so you can enjoy the flavor of this sandwich without the extra calories. Add additional vegetable toppings as desired and top with low-carbohydrate condiments like mustard and hot sauce. If you can tolerate bread items, feel free to use a high-fiber, high-protein, and low-carbohydrate wrap.

1 tablespoon extra-virgin olive oil

8 ounces stir-fry beef pieces

½ cup sliced yellow onion

¼ teaspoon salt

4 ounces Swiss cheese (4 slices)

4 romaine lettuce leaves

8 thin tomato slices

Serving Recommendations
GENERAL: about 1 full serving

1. In a large skillet, heat the oil over medium heat. Add the beef, onion, and salt and cook for 5 to 7 minutes, stirring frequently with tongs, until the beef is browned and onion is slightly translucent.

2. Reduce the heat to low and place the Swiss cheese slices on top of the beef. Place the lid on the skillet and cook for an additional minute to melt the cheese. Remove the beef and onion from the skillet and place in the center of the lettuce wraps.

3. Top the sandwiches with tomato slices.

STORAGE TIP: Store leftover beef in an airtight container and refrigerate for up to 3 days or freeze for up to 3 months. You can reheat the frozen beef in a skillet coated with nonstick cooking spray over medium heat for about 5 minutes or so. Prep new vegetables and cheese slices at time of serving if eating reheated leftovers.

PER SERVING (2 OUNCES BEEF, 1-OUNCE CHEESE, 2 SLICES TOMATO + 1 ROMAINE LETTUCE LEAF): Calories: 227; Protein: 20g; Fat: 15g; Carbohydrates: 4g; Fiber: 1g; Sugar: 1g; Sodium: 237mg

Simple Beef-and-Veggie Soup

SERVES 4 / PREP TIME: 5 MINUTES / COOK TIME: 35 MINUTES

Sometimes you just crave a hot cup of soup. The problem is that many soup recipes can take hours to make, which can be a turnoff and perhaps lead you to processed versions full of sodium and preservatives. Fortunately, this simple beef-and-veggie soup recipe takes less than 40 minutes, so you can satisfy your soup craving before you know it. If desired, add more veggies to the soup and add less bouillon to taste (or for lower sodium content).

1 tablespoon extra-virgin olive oil

2 cups peeled, chopped carrot

1 cup chopped yellow onion

3 cups water

3 teaspoons powdered beef bouillon

1 teaspoon garlic powder

Nonstick cooking spray

8 ounces lean ground beef

Serving Recommendations

PUREE: ¼ cup to ½ cup

SOFT FOODS: ½ cup to 1 cup

GENERAL: 1 to 2 cups

1. In a medium pot, heat the oil over medium heat. Cook the carrot and onion for 5 to 7 minutes, stirring frequently, until the onion is translucent.

2. Add the water, bouillon, and garlic powder. Simmer for about 5 minutes, stirring occasionally, to allow the flavors to develop.

3. While the broth simmers, heat a small skillet coated with nonstick cooking spray over medium heat. Place the beef in skillet and cook for 5 minutes, or until beef is no longer pink. Remove from the heat and place the beef in the pot with the vegetables and broth.

4. Reduce the heat to medium-low and simmer the soup for 20 minutes, or until the carrot has softened. Remove from heat and enjoy.

STORAGE TIP: Store leftovers in an airtight container and refrigerate for up to 3 days or freeze for up to 4 months.

PER SERVING (1 CUP): Calories: 175; Protein: 13g; Fat: 8g; Carbohydrates: 12g; Fiber: 3g; Sugar: 5g; Sodium: 474mg

Beef and Butternut Squash Stew

SERVES 4 / PREP TIME: 5 MINUTES / COOK TIME: 35 MINUTES

Beef stew is a comfort food favorite, especially on a cold winter's day. However, this type of thick and rich stew can contain a lot of sodium, fat, and calories. This version is rich in flavor, but lower in sodium and fat than restaurant versions or store-bought brands. And as a bonus, it only takes about 35 minutes to make.

1 tablespoon extra-virgin olive oil

1½ cups cubed butternut squash

1 cup chopped yellow onion

3 cups water

2 tablespoons cornstarch

3 teaspoons powdered beef bouillon

1 teaspoon garlic powder

Nonstick cooking spray

12 ounces lean ground beef

Serving Recommendations

PUREE: ¼ cup to ½ cup

SOFT FOODS: ½ cup to 1 cup

GENERAL: about 1 to 2 cups

1. In a medium pot, heat the oil over medium heat. Cook the butternut squash and onion for 5 to 7 minutes, stirring frequently, until the onion is translucent.

2. In a small bowl, mix the water and cornstarch to make a slurry. Add the slurry to the pot, stirring while pouring to ensure you transfer as much cornstarch as possible to the soup. Add the bouillon and garlic powder. Simmer for about 5 minutes, stirring occasionally.

3. While the broth simmers, coat a small skillet with nonstick cooking spray and heat over medium heat. Place the beef in the skillet and cook for 5 minutes, or until the beef is no longer pink. Remove from the heat and place the beef in the pot.

4. Reduce the heat to medium-low and simmer the soup for about 20 minutes, or until the squash has softened and the broth has thickened. Remove from the heat and enjoy.

STORAGE TIP: Store leftovers in an airtight container and refrigerate for up to 3 days or freeze for up to 4 months.

PER SERVING (1 CUP): Calories: 237; Protein: 19g; Fat: 10g; Carbohydrates: 18g; Fiber: 3g; Sugar: 3g; Sodium: 452mg

Lettuce Wrap Beef Tacos

SERVES 4 / PREP TIME: 5 MINUTES / COOK TIME: 15 MINUTES

Taco Tuesday is everyone's favorite night of the week, but it can also be a calorie- and fat-laden evening when celebrated with the traditional taco fillings and toppings. This lettuce wrap taco recipe, made with cauliflower rice and other heart-healthy vegetables, calls for nonfat Greek yogurt instead of sour cream, and makes taco night a healthy meal you can have anytime. You can find riced cauliflower, fresh or frozen, at most grocery stores.

1 tablespoon extra-virgin olive oil

8 ounces lean ground beef

1 cup chopped yellow onion

1 cup cauliflower rice

¼ cup water

1 teaspoon garlic powder

1 teaspoon ground cumin

¼ teaspoon salt

4 iceberg lettuce leaves

½ cup avocado

4 tablespoons nonfat plain Greek yogurt

Hot sauce *(optional)*

Serving Recommendations

SOFT FOODS: ½ cup to 1 cup

GENERAL: 1 to 2 cups

1. In a large skillet, heat the oil over medium heat. Cook the beef and onion for 5 to 7 minutes, stirring frequently, until the onion is translucent.

2. Add the cauliflower rice, water, garlic powder, cumin, and salt. Cover with a lid and let the cauliflower steam for 5 to 7 minutes until softened, lifting the lid to stir about every 30 seconds.

3. Remove from the heat and spoon the mixture into each lettuce leaf. Top each taco with 2 tablespoons of avocado and 1 tablespoon of nonfat Greek yogurt. Enjoy warm, topped with hot sauce, if desired.

STORAGE TIP: Store the leftover beef mixture in an airtight container and refrigerate for up to 3 days or freeze for up to 4 months.

PER SERVING (¾ CUP TACO MIXTURE): Calories: 185; Protein: 15g; Fat: 10g; Carbohydrates: 8g; Fiber: 4g; Sugar: 4g; Sodium: 203mg

Zucchini Noodles and Beef Marinara

SERVES 4 / PREP TIME: 5 MINUTES / COOK TIME: 25 MINUTES

Spaghetti with meat sauce is a quick and tasty meal for those busy days when you just don't feel like cooking, but a quick swap of zucchini noodles and lean beef can cut calories, carbohydrates, and fat content without sacrificing flavor. Prep the zucchini and onion the night before to make this quickly. If you like a creamier sauce, add a few tablespoons of plain, unsweetened nonfat Greek yogurt.

3 tablespoons extra-virgin olive oil, divided

8 ounces lean ground beef

3 cups canned diced tomatoes, drained

1 cup diced onion

2 teaspoons garlic powder

1 teaspoon chopped fresh basil

1 teaspoon paprika

2 teaspoons Italian seasoning

½ teaspoon salt

2 medium zucchinis, peeled vertically into flat, wide strips

1. In a large skillet, heat 1 tablespoon of oil over medium heat. Cook the ground beef, stirring frequently, for about 5 minutes, until browned. Remove the beef from the skillet and place in a small bowl. Set aside.

2. In the same skillet, heat 1 tablespoon of oil. Add the tomato and onion to the skillet and stir occasionally, about every 30 seconds. Cook for 5 to 7 minutes, or until the onion is translucent.

3. Add the garlic powder, Italian seasoning, basil, paprika, and salt to the tomato and onion. Remove from heat and blend mixture in a blender on low for about 15 seconds or until smooth. Transfer the sauce back to the skillet and add in the cooked beef. Place on low heat and simmer.

4. In a separate skillet over medium heat, heat the remaining 1 tablespoon of oil. Cook the zucchini noodles for 3 to 5 minutes, stirring frequently or until softened.

5. Serve the zucchini noodles topped with the beef sauce.

> **STORAGE TIP:** Store the beef marinara sauce in an airtight container and refrigerate for up to 3 days or freeze for up to 4 months. Store leftover zucchini noodles in an airtight container in the refrigerator for 2 to 3 days. The marinara sauce and the zucchini noodles can be reheated in a skillet over medium heat for a few minutes before serving.

PER SERVING (¾ TO 1 CUP SAUCE + ¾ CUP ZUCCHINI NOODLES):
Calories: 234; Protein: 14g; Fat: 15g; Carbohydrates: 13g; Fiber: 3g; Sugar: 7g; Sodium: 547mg

Serving Recommendations
SOFT FOODS: ½ cup sauce and ½ cup zucchini noodles

GENERAL: 1 to 2 full servings of sauce and zucchini noodles, depending on daily calorie needs

Brown Sugar, Beef, and Broccoli Stir-Fry

SERVES 4 / PREP TIME: 5 MINUTES / COOK TIME: 15 MINUTES

On the weekends or busy weeknights, you may enjoy ordering takeout meals like beef and broccoli. Although beef and broccoli stir-fry looks healthy since it's not fried, it's still high in sodium and sugar from the sauce that's used to flavor it. However, you can still enjoy the taste of beef and broccoli without the extra sodium and sugar with this quick meal option. If you want more flavor, add more coconut aminos since this soy sauce alternative is low in sodium.

1 tablespoon extra-virgin olive oil

8 ounces stir-fry beef pieces

Nonstick cooking spray

2 cups chopped broccoli florets

1 cup sliced yellow onion

2 tablespoons coconut aminos

2 tablespoons brown sugar

½ tablespoon soy sauce

Serving Recommendations
GENERAL: 1 to 2 full servings, depending on daily calorie needs

1. In a large skillet, heat the oil over medium heat. Cook the beef, stirring frequently with tongs, until browned, about 5 minutes.

2. Transfer the beef to a small bowl. Set aside.

3. Spray the skillet with cooking spray. Place the broccoli and onion in the skillet and stir occasionally, about every 30 seconds. Cook for 5 to 7 minutes or until the onion is translucent.

4. Add the coconut aminos, brown sugar, soy sauce, and cooked beef. Mix well.

5. Remove the beef and broccoli from the heat and serve.

STORAGE TIP: Store leftovers in an airtight container and refrigerate for up to 3 days or freeze for up to 4 months.

PER SERVING (2 OUNCES BEEF + ¾ CUP VEGETABLES): Calories: 152; Protein: 15g; Fat: 6g; Carbohydrates: 10g; Fiber: 1g; Sugar: 7g; Sodium: 294mg

Tomato-Parmesan Beef Burgers

SERVES 4 / PREP TIME: 10 MINUTES / COOK TIME: 15 MINUTES

You may be familiar with chicken Parmesan, but you likely have not had a Parmesan burger before. This twist on the Italian restaurant classic gives you a juicy burger with Parmesan melted inside and fresh, warmed tomatoes on top. Enjoy alone or on your favorite lettuce or other low-carbohydrate sandwich wrap.

1 tablespoon extra-virgin olive oil

½ cup chopped yellow onion

8 ounces lean ground beef

4 tablespoons almond flour

4 tablespoons shredded Parmesan cheese

1 teaspoon garlic powder

1 teaspoon Italian seasoning

¼ teaspoon salt

1 large egg

Nonstick cooking spray

1 cup canned diced tomatoes, drained

Serving Recommendations

SOFT FOODS: 1 burger and ¼ cup diced tomatoes

GENERAL: 1 to 2 burgers and ¼ to ½ cup tomatoes, depending on daily calorie needs

1. In a large skillet, heat the oil over medium heat. Cook the onion for 5 to 7 minutes, stirring frequently, until it is translucent. Remove from the heat.

2. In a medium mixing bowl, mix the ground beef, almond flour, Parmesan cheese, garlic powder, Italian seasoning, salt, and cooked onion together with a fork until well incorporated.

3. In a small bowl, beat the egg, then add to the ground beef mixture and combine well. Form the meat mixture into 4 patties with your hands.

4. Spray the same skillet with nonstick cooking spray and place over medium heat. Place the patties in the skillet. Cook for 3 to 4 minutes on each side, until browned. After you flip the burgers, add the diced tomatoes to warm. Move the tomatoes around the skillet frequently to prevent burning.

5. Once the burgers are done, remove from heat and serve topped with tomatoes.

> **STORAGE TIP:** Store leftover burgers in an airtight container and refrigerate for up to 3 days or freeze for up to 6 months.

PER SERVING (1 [2–2 ½ OUNCE] BURGER + ¼ CUP DICED TOMATOES): Calories: 226; Protein: 18g; Fat: 14g; Carbohydrates: 7g; Fiber: 2g; Sugar: 3g; Sodium: 412mg

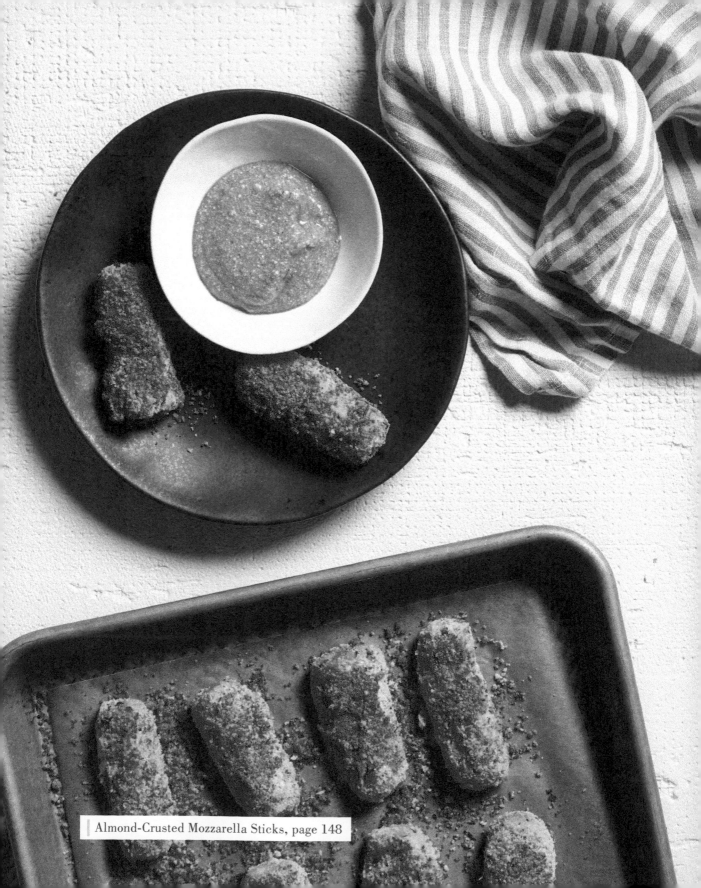

Almond-Crusted Mozzarella Sticks, page 148

CHAPTER EIGHT

Snacks and Treats

Garlic-Parmesan Cheesy Chips

MAKES 12 CHIPS / PREP TIME: 2 MINUTES, PLUS 20 MINUTES TO COOL / COOK TIME: 7 MINUTES

The salty, crunchy taste of chips can be satisfying, but also not so good for your health. Fortunately, there's a tasty alternative to such salty snacks that provides plenty of protein, as well as less sodium and fat. These chips may not provide a crisp crunch, but can act as a savory spoon for your favorite dip, salsa, or other sauce.

¼ cup shredded
  Parmesan cheese
¼ cup shredded sharp
  Cheddar cheese
¼ teaspoon garlic powder
Dash salt

Serving Recommendations
SOFT FOODS: 2 to 4 chips
GENERAL: 4 to 6 chips (or more as tolerated depending on daily calorie needs)

1. Preheat the oven to 400°F. Line a large baking sheet with parchment paper.

2. In a medium mixing bowl, combine the Parmesan cheese, Cheddar cheese, garlic powder, and salt. Mix well.

3. Place 2 teaspoons of the cheese mixture about an inch or two apart on the baking sheet, making about 12 chips.

4. Bake for 5 to 7 minutes, or until the chips are golden brown around the edges.

5. Remove from the oven and let sit for 15 to 20 minutes, or until the chips start to crisp. Enjoy.

STORAGE TIP: Place leftover chips in a paper towel–lined storage container. The chips will store well at room temperature for 2 to 3 days.

PER SERVING (6 CHIPS): Calories: 98; Protein: 8g; Fat: 7g; Carbohydrate: 1g; Fiber: 0g; Sugar: 0g; Sodium: 333mg

Cheesy Baked Radish Chips

MAKES 1 CUP / PREP TIME: 5 MINUTES / COOK TIME: 35 MINUTES

Potato chips are a classic salty snack to enjoy alone or with your favorite lunch item. However, potatoes are high in carbohydrates and most chips can be very salty and not so heart healthy. But it's not impossible to have a healthy chip. These baked radish chips provide a cheesy flavor with high protein nutritional yeast and use low-carbohydrate radishes instead of potatoes.

1 cup thinly sliced radishes (2 bunches radishes)

1 tablespoon extra-virgin olive oil

3 tablespoons nutritional yeast flakes

¼ teaspoon salt

Dash freshly ground black pepper *(optional)*

Serving Recommendations
SOFT FOODS: ¼ to ½ cup chips
GENERAL: ½ to 1 cup chips

1. Preheat the oven to 375°F. Line a baking sheet with parchment paper.

2. Place the radishes into a small bowl and toss in the oil.

3. In a small cup, mix the nutritional yeast, salt, and pepper (if using).

4. Place the oil-coated radish slices onto the prepared baking sheet in a single layer and sprinkle the nutritional yeast mixture lightly onto each slice.

5. Bake for about 15 minutes, then flip the chips and bake for another 15 minutes. Remove crispy chips, then continue to bake any remaining chips for a few minutes more at a time, until crispy and golden brown.

6. Serve and enjoy alone or with your favorite low-carbohydrate dip.

STORAGE TIP: Store in a paper towel–lined container at room temperature. Consume within 2 to 3 days for best freshness.

PER SERVING (½ CUP CHIPS): Calories: 99; Protein: 5g; Fat: 7g; Carbohydrates: 4g; Fiber: 2g; Sugar: 0g; Sodium: 313mg

Savory Cheese Biscuits

MAKES 8 BISCUITS / PREP TIME: 5 MINUTES / COOK TIME: 15 MINUTES

Biscuits go great with soup, chili, or any comfort food classic meal. However, they are typically high in carbohydrates, so they aren't ideal for a post-op bariatric eating plan. But if you replace the wheat flour with almond flour and shredded cheese, these savory biscuits can give you the taste of biscuits without the carbohydrates. If you are trying to watch your fat content, then it may help you to cut the serving size down to 1 biscuit or add less cheese.

1 cup almond flour
¼ cup shredded
   Parmesan cheese
¼ cup shredded
   Cheddar cheese
2 teaspoons
   baking powder
2 teaspoons garlic powder
½ teaspoon salt
2 large eggs

Serving Recommendations
SOFT FOODS: ½ to 1 biscuit
GENERAL: 1 to 2 biscuits

1. Preheat the oven to 350°F. Line a large baking sheet with parchment paper and set aside.

2. In a large bowl, add the almond flour, Parmesan cheese, Cheddar cheese, baking powder, garlic powder, and salt. Mix well. Add the eggs and combine.

3. Scoop a heaping tablespoon of the mixture onto the baking sheet. Using a spatula, flatten the batter slightly into about 2-inch circles. Repeat, placing biscuits about an inch apart. This should yield 8 small biscuits.

4. Bake for 15 minutes, or until the top of biscuits is slightly golden brown. Serve warm.

STORAGE TIP: Store the biscuits in an airtight container at room temperature for 1 to 2 days or in the refrigerator for about 1 week. Reheat refrigerated biscuits for 15 to 20 seconds in the microwave. You can also freeze leftover biscuits in a freezer bag for up to 3 months and reheat for 20 minutes at 300°F.

PER SERVING (2 BISCUITS): Calories: 275; Protein: 15g; Fat: 23g; Carbohydrates: 8g; Fiber: 3g; Sugar: 1g; Sodium: 447mg

Italian Herb Muffins

MAKES 4 MUFFINS / PREP TIME: 5 MINUTES / COOK TIME: 12 MINUTES

Dinner rolls can be a terrific addition to mealtime to dip into your soup or enjoy with butter. However, classic dinner rolls don't provide much nutrition to your day, just carbohydrates. This Italian herb muffin offers savory flavor in a delicious bread substitute with plenty of protein to boot. These muffins taste great alone or with a spread of butter, or they can be used to create savory sliders with your favorite protein choice.

Nonstick cooking spray
8 tablespoons almond flour
¼ cup shredded
  Parmesan cheese
1 large egg
1 teaspoon garlic powder
1 teaspoon Italian
  seasoning
1 teaspoon baking powder
¼ teaspoon salt

Serving Recommendations
SOFT FOODS: ½ to 1 muffin

GENERAL: 1 to 2 muffins (or as tolerated; depending on your daily calorie needs)

1. Preheat the oven to 350°F. Line a muffin pan with 4 cupcake liners and spray the liners with nonstick cooking spray.

2. In a large mixing bowl, combine the almond flour, Parmesan cheese, egg, garlic powder, Italian seasoning, baking powder, and salt. Mix well until fully incorporated.

3. Scoop heaping tablespoons of the mixture into the lined cups until all the batter is used.

4. Bake for 12 minutes or until golden brown on the tops. Enjoy warm.

STORAGE TIP: Store the muffins in an airtight container at room temperature for 1 to 2 days or refrigerate for about 1 week. Reheat refrigerated muffins for 15 to 20 seconds in the microwave. You can also freeze leftover muffins in a freezer bag for up to 3 months and reheat for 20 minutes at 300°F.

PER SERVING (1 MUFFIN): Calories: 128; Protein: 7g; Fat: 10g; Carbohydrates: 5g; Fiber: 2g; Sugar: 1g; Sodium: 217mg

Cheesy Cauliflower Tots

SERVES 4 / PREP TIME: 5 MINUTES / COOK TIME: 15 MINUTES

Tater tots are a nostalgic food that you may remember from your grade school days. But you may not eat them anymore unless you're stealing from a kid's plate since they're usually full of carbohydrates and fat. However, if you start to crave a tot or two, this cauliflower rice tot recipe will provide a lower fat and lower carbohydrate alternative you don't have to ditch from your daily eating plan. These tots pair well with Creamy Marinara Dipping Sauce (page 165).

1 cup cauliflower rice

½ cup almond flour

½ cup shredded mozzarella cheese

1 large egg

1 tablespoon cornstarch

¼ teaspoon salt

Serving Recommendations

SOFT FOODS: 4 tots

GENERAL: 4 to 8 tots (or as tolerated; depending on your daily calorie needs)

1. Preheat the oven to 400°F. Line a large baking sheet with parchment paper and set aside.

2. In a large mixing bowl, combine the cauliflower rice, almond flour, mozzarella cheese, egg, cornstarch, and salt. Mix well until fully incorporated.

3. Scoop heaping tablespoons of the mixture onto the baking sheet about an inch apart until all the batter is used. This recipe should make about 16 tots.

4. Bake for 13 to 15 minutes, until crispy and golden brown. Serve and enjoy.

> **STORAGE TIP:** Store the tots in an airtight container in the refrigerator for up to 1 week or in the freezer for up to 1 month. Reheat frozen tots at 350°F for about 15 minutes.

PER SERVING (4 TOTS): Calories: 152; Protein: 9g; Fat: 11g; Carbohydrates: 6g; Fiber: 2g; Sugar: 1g; Sodium: 253mg

Mozzarella Mushroom Caps

MAKES 12 CAPS / PREP TIME: 5 MINUTES / COOK TIME: 20 MINUTES

Whether it's happy hour, a party, or just a bite before dinner, appetizers are created to spark your appetite before mealtime. These mozzarella mushroom caps provide a perfect balance of fresh veggie and creamy cheese to give you a healthy alternative to typical fried appetizer favorites. Feel free to substitute the mozzarella with your favorite cheese for a different flavor if you like.

12 white mushroom caps
4 ounces fresh
  mozzarella pearls
2 tablespoons almond flour
1 tablespoon
  whipped butter
½ teaspoon garlic powder
Dash salt

Serving Recommendations
SOFT FOODS: 1 to
2 mushroom caps

GENERAL: 3 mushroom caps
(or as tolerated; depending
on your daily calorie needs)

1. Preheat the oven to 350°F. Line a baking sheet with parchment paper.

2. Wash the mushrooms and carefully remove the cap from each one. Place the mushrooms onto the lined baking sheet.

3. Place about three mozzarella pearls (about 1 tablespoon) in each mushroom cap.

4. In a small bowl, mix the almond flour, whipped butter, garlic powder, and salt. Sprinkle the mixture on top of each mushroom cap.

5. Bake for about 20 minutes or until the cheese has melted. Enjoy warm.

STORAGE TIP: Store leftovers in an airtight container in the refrigerator for up to 3 days.

PER SERVING (3 MUSHROOM CAPS): Calories: 117; Protein: 8g; Fat: 9g; Carbohydrates: 4g; Fiber: 1g; Sugar: 0.25g; Sodium: 141mg

Almond-Crusted Mozzarella Sticks

MAKES 6 STICKS / PREP TIME: 10 MINUTES, PLUS 2 HOURS TO FREEZE / COOK TIME: 6 MINUTES

Mozzarella sticks are a fried appetizer classic at many restaurants and bars but are covered in fat- and carbohydrate-laden batter. However, the baked form of this snack is just as yummy without all the excess calories, sodium, and fat. Olive oil is brushed on the sticks before cooking to create the golden crust, but if you need to lower the fat, cooking spray can be used instead. Pair these with Creamy Marinara Dipping Sauce (page 165).

1 tablespoon cornstarch

8 tablespoons almond flour

½ teaspoon Italian seasoning

¼ teaspoon salt

2 large eggs

6 (1-ounce) light mozzarella sticks

1 tablespoon extra-virgin olive oil

Serving Recommendations
SOFT FOODS:
2 mozzarella sticks

GENERAL: 4 to 6 mozzarella sticks

1. Place the cornstarch on a small plate. On a separate small plate, mix the almond flour, Italian seasoning, and salt. Beat the eggs in a small bowl and place between the two plates.

2. Cut the mozzarella sticks in half. Lightly coat each mozzarella stick in cornstarch, then dip and coat in the egg, and then coat well in the almond flour mixture. Coat each mozzarella piece well with the batter to enclose the cheese in the mixture so it doesn't spread onto the baking sheet while baking. Place each coated mozzarella piece on a large plate. Repeat until all the mozzarella pieces are coated.

3. Cover the plate with plastic wrap and place the mozzarella sticks in the freezer for about 2 hours.

4. Preheat the oven to 400°F. Line a baking sheet with parchment paper.

5. Place the mozzarella pieces about 1-inch apart on the baking sheet. Using a basting brush, coat each side of each mozzarella piece lightly with the oil.

6. Bake for 4 to 6 minutes, until the cheese starts to bubble, and the crust starts to turn slightly golden. Watch closely to make sure the cheese does not start to spread. Enjoy warm.

STORAGE TIP: Store mozzarella sticks in an airtight container in the refrigerator for up to 1 week or in the freezer for up to 1 month. Reheat frozen sticks in the microwave on high for about 20 to 30 seconds.

PER SERVING (2 MOZZARELLA STICKS): Calories: 182; Protein: 11g; Fat: 15g; Carbohydrates: 4g; Fiber: 1g; Sugar: 1g; Sodium: 311mg

Almond Light-as-Air Cookies

MAKES 8 COOKIES / PREP TIME: 5 MINUTES / COOK TIME: 10 MINUTES

Cookies are the center of many special events in life such as holidays, birthday parties, and social events. But cookies can also be full of sugar and carbohydrates that are not a balanced part of a healthy diet. These light-as-air cookies provide a buttery and subtly sweet flavor that tastes great alone or pairs well with your favorite low-sugar jam.

8 tablespoons almond flour

1 tablespoon low-sugar vanilla whey protein powder

1 tablespoon whipped butter

2 teaspoons vanilla extract

1 teaspoon baking powder

1 teaspoon finely granulated pure cane sugar

½ teaspoon stevia or no-calorie sweetener

¼ teaspoon salt

Serving Recommendations

SOFT FOODS: 1 to 2 cookies

GENERAL: 2 to 3 cookies (or as tolerated; depending on your daily calorie needs)

1. Preheat the oven to 350°F. Line a large baking sheet with parchment paper.

2. In a large bowl, combine the almond flour, protein powder, whipped butter, vanilla extract, baking powder, sugar, stevia, and salt and mix well until fully incorporated.

3. Scoop heaping tablespoons of the mixture onto the baking sheet about an inch apart. Using a spatula, flatten the batter slightly into about 2-inch circles. This should yield 8 cookies.

4. Bake for 7 to 9 minutes, or until the edges of cookies are slightly golden brown. Keep a close eye on the cookies since as soon as this happens, you will want to remove the cookies from the oven to prevent overcooking.

5. Allow the cookies to cool slightly before serving.

STORAGE TIP: Store the cookies in an airtight container at room temperature for up to 3 days or refrigerate for up to 1 week.

PER SERVING (2 COOKIES): Calories: 117; Protein: 6g; Fat: 9g; Carbohydrates: 5g; Fiber: 2g; Sugar: 2g; Sodium: 288mg

Strawberry Gelatin Tea

SERVES 1 / PREP TIME: 5 MINUTES / COOK TIME: 5 MINUTES

A hot cup of tea can help your body and mind relax after a long and busy day. Although tea provides antioxidants, it doesn't add protein to your daily intake if you're trying to get as much protein as possible in every bite and sip. This gelatin tea brings the fresh flavor of strawberries in a protein-rich gelatin tea form.

½ cup frozen sliced
strawberries

¼ teaspoon stevia or
no-calorie sweetener

½ cup hot water

2 tablespoons plain
gelatin powder

Serving Recommendations

LIQUID: 2 to 4 tablespoons

PUREE: ¼ to ½ cup

SOFT FOODS: ½ cup to 1 cup
(about 1 serving)

GENERAL: 1 to 2 servings, as tolerated

1. In a small saucepan, cook the strawberries over medium heat for 3 minutes, stirring frequently, until softened.

2. Stir in the stevia. Remove the pan from the heat and set aside.

3. Pour the hot water into a mug. Mix in the gelatin powder a bit at a time while continuously stirring with a fork. Keep stirring as you add in the cooked strawberries.

4. Blend the mixture in a blender for about 30 seconds, until frothy.

5. Pour into a mug. Sip once cooled and enjoy as a tea within about 15 minutes or so before it starts to set.

COOKING TIP: If you prefer, set the gelatin in the refrigerator for about an hour or so to enjoy as a gelatin dessert.

PER SERVING (¾ CUP OR 12 TABLESPOONS): Calories: 89; Protein: 12g; Fat: 0g; Carbohydrates: 10g; Fiber: 2g; Sugar: 5g; Sodium: 47mg

Subtly Sweet Coconut Milk "Flan"

SERVES 1 / PREP TIME: 5 MINUTES, PLUS 1 HOUR TO CHILL / COOK TIME: 5 MINUTES

Are you sick of eating gelatin with artificial dyes, colorings, and a chemical aftertaste of fruit flavors? If so, then you'll be refreshed to taste this subtly sweet vanilla and coconut low-sugar, flan-like gelatin dessert. If you want to take this dessert a step further, feel free to top with sugar-free whipped topping.

½ cup light unsweetened coconut milk

2 teaspoons vanilla extract

1 teaspoon stevia or no-calorie sweetener

1 tablespoon (1 packet) plain gelatin powder

Serving Recommendations
PUREE: 4 to 6 tablespoons
SOFT FOODS: 1 full serving
GENERAL: 1 to 2 full servings

1. In a small saucepan, heat the coconut milk for 1 to 2 minutes, then sprinkle in the vanilla extract and stevia and stir to dissolve.

2. Sprinkle in the gelatin while stirring constantly to dissolve the gelatin completely. Remove from the heat.

3. Transfer the mixture to a blender and blend for about 30 seconds or so, until frothy. Pour into a small jar or mug.

4. Allow the dessert to set in the refrigerator for about an hour to firm.

5. Serve and enjoy.

INGREDIENT TIP: If you prefer a sweeter taste, add a bit more sweetener to the recipe or substitute sugar-free flavored syrup instead. If you prefer a more mousse-like texture, then double the coconut milk in the recipe, while keeping the gelatin measurement the same. If you double the milk, it's important to note that it will take 2 hours to set and the carbohydrates will increase by 4 grams, making carbohydrates higher than the protein in this recipe.

PER SERVING (6 TABLESPOONS): Calories: 130; Protein: 6g; Fat: 7g; Carbohydrates: 5g; Fiber: 0g; Sugar: 3g; Sodium: 51mg

Chia Chocolate Pudding

SERVES 1 / PREP TIME: 5 MINUTES, PLUS 2 TO 8 HOURS TO CHILL

Pudding is a creamy snack classic that is usually made primarily from milk and sugar. But if you're trying to make your desserts delicious and nutritious, chia pudding is a healthy option. The chia seeds provide fiber and healthy fats, while the Greek yogurt and whey protein are a rich source of protein. A dash of cocoa powder makes this pudding alternative enough to satisfy your chocolate cravings any time of day.

½ cup unsweetened almond milk

½ cup nonfat plain Greek yogurt

2 tablespoons chia seeds

1 tablespoon vanilla whey protein

1 teaspoon unsweetened cocoa powder

½ teaspoon stevia or no-calorie sweetener

1. In a canning jar, combine the almond milk, yogurt, chia seeds, whey protein, cocoa powder, and stevia.

2. Seal with lid and let sit in refrigerator overnight.

3. Enjoy straight from the jar, or in a separate bowl if you are consuming a smaller serving.

PER SERVING (1¼ CUP): Calories: 257; Protein: 25g; Fat: 12g; Carbohydrates: 21g; Fiber: 11g; Sugar: 5g; Sodium: 122mg

Serving Recommendations

PUREE: ¼ to ½ cup (4 to 8 tablespoons)

SOFT FOODS: ½ cup to 1 cup (8 to 16 tablespoons)

GENERAL: ¾ cup to 1 full serving

Simply Vanilla Frozen Greek Yogurt

MAKES 4 CUPS / PREP TIME: 5 MINUTES, PLUS 8 HOURS TO FREEZE

Ice cream may be one of the top things most people miss when starting a healthy eating plan, but it doesn't have to be. This recipe takes the classic taste of vanilla ice cream and makes it from the protein-rich and creamy content of Greek yogurt. Enjoy on its own or pair with your favorite low-carbohydrate fruit, like berries.

4 cups nonfat plain
  Greek yogurt

4 tablespoons vanilla whey
  protein powder

4 tablespoons
  vanilla extract

4 teaspoons stevia or
  no-calorie sweetener

Serving Recommendations

PUREE: ¼ cup to ½ cup

SOFT FOODS: ½ cup to 1 cup

GENERAL: 1 to 1½ cups (or as tolerated; depending on your daily calorie needs)

1. In a large bowl or loaf pan, combine the yogurt, protein powder, vanilla extract, and stevia.

2. Cover and freeze overnight or for at least 8 hours.

3. About an hour before serving, set in the refrigerator to thaw slightly. Serve and enjoy.

STORAGE TIP: Freeze for up to 2 months in a freezer-safe container.

PER SERVING (1 CUP): Calories: 183; Protein: 28g; Fat: 1g; Carbohydrates: 12g; Fiber: 1g; Sugar: 8g; Sodium: 96mg

Chocolate and Peanut Butter Cupcakes

MAKES 6 CUPCAKES / PREP TIME: 5 MINUTES / COOK TIME: 15 MINUTES

Chocolate and peanut butter make a decadent combination for dessert, but unfortunately they are usually full of sugar and carbohydrates. If you want to have your cake and eat it, too, this cupcake is for you. A combination of almond flour, peanut butter powder, and cocoa powder create a delicious dessert for any day of the week.

Nonstick cooking spray

½ cup sugar-free peanut butter powder

2 large eggs

2 tablespoons vanilla whey protein powder

2 tablespoons unsweetened cocoa powder

2 tablespoons unsweetened almond milk

2 tablespoons coconut flour

2 teaspoons stevia or no-calorie sweetener

1 teaspoon baking powder

Dash salt

Serving Recommendations
SOFT FOODS: ½ to 1 cupcake

GENERAL: 1 to 2 cupcakes (or as tolerated; depending on your daily calorie needs)

1. Preheat the oven to 350°F. Line a cupcake pan with 6 cupcake liners and spray the liners with nonstick cooking spray. Set aside.

2. In a large bowl, combine the peanut butter powder, eggs, protein powder, cocoa powder, almond milk, coconut flour, stevia, baking powder, and salt and mix well to combine.

3. Scoop heaping tablespoons of the mixture into the cupcake liners to evenly fill the cups.

4. Bake for 13 to 15 minutes, or until a toothpick or butter knife inserted in the center of cupcake comes out clean.

5. Allow the cupcakes to cool completely before enjoying.

INGREDIENT TIP: You are welcome to substitute chocolate-flavored whey protein powder. If you do this, then do not add cocoa powder to the recipe.

STORAGE TIP: Store cupcakes in an airtight container at room temperature for up to 3 days or refrigerate for up to 1 week.

PER SERVING (1 CUPCAKE): Calories: 92; Protein: 10g; Fat: 4g; Carbohydrates: 7g; Fiber: 3g; Sugar: 2g; Sodium: 89mg

Cinnamon Cream Cheese–Filled Almond Cakes

MAKES 8 CAKES / PREP TIME: 5 MINUTES / COOK TIME: 10 MINUTES

A cannoli or crepe is a light and sweet dessert after a special dinner meal. But these sugary treats are just that: packed with lots of sugar. That doesn't mean similar dessert options are off-limits. This thin crepe-like almond pancake filled with cinnamon cream cheese tastes great, while cutting back on your sugar intake and increasing protein consumption during dessert.

For the pancakes

3 large eggs

3 tablespoons plain whipped cream cheese

2 tablespoons almond flour

1 tablespoon whipped butter, at room temperature

1 tablespoon cornstarch

½ teaspoon stevia or no-calorie sweetener

1 teaspoon vanilla extract

Dash salt

Nonstick cooking spray

For the filling

4 tablespoons whipped cream cheese

4 tablespoons nonfat plain Greek yogurt

1 teaspoon ground cinnamon

To make the pancakes

1. In a large mixing bowl, combine the eggs, cream cheese, coconut flour, whipped butter, cornstarch, stevia, vanilla extract, and salt and mix well.

2. Spray a large skillet with nonstick cooking spray and heat over medium heat. Scoop about 1 to 2 tablespoons of the pancake mixture onto the skillet and tilt the skillet to coat a large round cake shape (at least 4 inches in diameter).

3. Cook for about 45 seconds on the first side until the edges are slightly golden brown and bubbles form in the cake. Flip over and cook for an additional 20 to 30 seconds. Remove from skillet and repeat with rest of the batter. This recipe should make 7 or 8 pancakes.

To make the filling

4. In a medium mixing bowl, combine the cream cheese, yogurt, and cinnamon and mix well.

5. Scoop a heaping tablespoon of the filling in the center of each cake and spread over one side of the pancake. Starting from the bottom of the cake, roll into a cannoli shape. Repeat for the rest of the cakes and enjoy. Serve as is or with your favorite low-carbohydrate fruits like blueberries or sliced strawberries.

STORAGE TIP: Store almond cakes in an airtight container in the refrigerator for up to 3 days for best freshness.

PER SERVING (1 ALMOND CAKE + 1 TABLESPOON FILLING):
Calories: 71; Protein: 4g; Fat: 5g; Carbohydrates: 4g; Fiber: 1g; Sugar: 1g; Sodium: 96mg

Serving Recommendations
SOFT FOODS: ½ to 1 almond cake

GENERAL: 1 almond cake

Clockwise from Top Left: Avocado Mayo, page 160;
Creamy Marinara Dipping Sauce, page 165;
Blue Cheese and Yogurt Dressing, page 166;
Low-Carb Honey Mustard Yogurt Dressing, page 169

CHAPTER NINE

Homemade Staples

Avocado Mayo

MAKES ¾ CUP / PREP TIME: 5 MINUTES

If you enjoy your tuna or chicken salad sandwiches with a touch of moisture, but without too much unhealthy fat, you'll enjoy this refreshing alternative to mayonnaise. With a subtle seasoning and the natural flavor of avocado, this condiment can be used with just about any dish to add a touch of creaminess and flavor.

6 tablespoons mashed avocado (½ avocado)

⅓ cup nonfat plain Greek yogurt

¼ teaspoon garlic powder

¼ teaspoon salt

Serving Recommendations

LIQUID: 1 to 2 tablespoons

PUREE: 2 to 3 tablespoons

SOFT FOODS: 3 tablespoons

GENERAL: 4 tablespoons

1. In a medium mixing bowl, combine the avocado, yogurt, garlic powder, and salt and mix well.

2. If you prefer a creamier, smoother texture, place all the ingredients into a blender and blend for about 1 minute on low.

STORAGE TIP: Due to the rapid browning of avocado fruit, place the mayo in a tightly airtight container in your refrigerator and consume within 3 days.

PER SERVING (3 TABLESPOONS): Calories: 45; Protein: 3g; Fat: 3g; Carbohydrates: 3g (1 net gram); Fiber: 2g; Sugar: 1g; Sodium: 154mg

Citrus-Avocado Salad Dressing

MAKES ABOUT 1 CUP / PREP TIME: 5 MINUTES

Salad dressings can be full of fat and excess calories that can sabotage your healthy eating plan. And low-fat or fat-free dressings typically provide little in the way of satisfying flavor. However, this simple combination of avocado, lemon juice, yogurt, and spices creates a flavorful dressing that can enhance any meat, salad, or vegetable. Feel free to add a bit of ground black pepper or hot sauce for a spicier flavor.

¾ cup nonfat plain Greek yogurt

½ cup mashed avocado (½ avocado)

1 tablespoon freshly squeezed lemon juice

1 teaspoon dried or chopped fresh cilantro

1 teaspoon garlic powder

¼ teaspoon salt

1. In a medium mixing bowl, combine the yogurt, avocado, lemon juice, cilantro, garlic powder, and salt and mix well.

2. If you prefer a creamier, smoother texture, place all the ingredients into a blender and blend for about 1 minute on low.

STORAGE TIP: Store in an airtight container in the refrigerator for up to 3 days.

Serving Recommendations
LIQUID: 1 to 2 tablespoons
PUREE: 2 to 3 tablespoons
SOFT FOODS: 3 tablespoons
GENERAL: 4 tablespoons

PER SERVING (3 TABLESPOONS): Calories: 71; Protein: 5g; Fat: 4g; Carbohydrates: 4g; Fiber: <1g; Sugar: 1g; Sodium: 164mg

Vegan Garlic Cream Sauce

MAKES 1¼ CUPS / PREP TIME: 5 MINUTES

If you enjoy the savory taste of alfredo sauce but can't tolerate cream or don't eat dairy, try this tofu cream sauce. This vegan garlic cream sauce provides a creamy texture perfect for pasta, vegetables, or proteins. And compared to similar milk or cream-based sauces, this sauce recipe provides more protein and less fat.

1 cup diced firm tofu

2 tablespoons unsweetened almond milk

½ tablespoon garlic powder

¼ teaspoon salt

1. Add the tofu, almond milk, garlic powder, and salt to a blender.

2. Blend on low for 30 to 60 seconds for a creamy, smooth texture.

> **STORAGE TIP:** Store the cream sauce in an airtight container in the refrigerator for up to 5 days. This sauce can be enjoyed warmed or cold.

Serving Recommendations

LIQUID: 1 to 2 tablespoons

PUREE: 2 to 3 tablespoons

SOFT FOODS: 3 tablespoons

GENERAL: 4 tablespoons

PER SERVING (¼ CUP): Calories: 46; Protein: 4g; Fat: 2g; Carbohydrates: 2g; Fiber: 1g; Sugar: 0g; Sodium: 126mg

Greek Yogurt Caesar Dressing

MAKES ½ CUP / PREP TIME: 5 MINUTES

Caesar salad is a simple and savory favorite in many restaurants as a starter to meals or entrée with protein. But the dressing alone is full of fat and calories that can make your typically healthy salad a calorie-laden one. This Greek yogurt–based salad dressing takes the flavors of Caesar salad and puts them in a low-fat version that reduces calories without reducing deliciousness.

½ cup nonfat plain Greek yogurt

½ cup shredded Parmesan cheese

Juice of 1 small lemon (2 tablespoons)

1 tablespoon extra-virgin olive oil

1 teaspoon garlic powder

¼ teaspoon salt

Dash freshly ground black pepper

1. Add the yogurt, Parmesan cheese, lemon juice, oil, garlic powder, salt, and pepper to a blender.

2. Blend on low for about 30 seconds or until smooth.

> **STORAGE TIP:** Store the dressing in an airtight container in the refrigerator for up to 7 days for maximum freshness.

PER SERVING (2 TABLESPOONS): Calories: 100; Protein: 7g; Fat: 7g; Carbohydrates: 3g; Fiber: <1g; Sugar: 1g; Sodium: 382mg

Serving Recommendations
LIQUID: 1 to 2 tablespoons
PUREE: 2 to 3 tablespoons
SOFT FOODS: 3 tablespoons
GENERAL: 4 tablespoons

Creamy Peanut Sauce

MAKES ¾ CUP / PREP TIME: 5 MINUTES

In Thai cuisine, peanut sauce is often used in dishes like Pad Thai or as a dipping sauce for skewered meat or satay. This peanut sauce recreates that same taste using ingredients you may have at home already and adds extra protein to your meal through the use of tofu as the sauce base. Use this sauce in stir-fry dishes, over your favorite proteins, or chilled as a unique salad dressing alternative.

⅔ cup cubed firm tofu

2 tablespoons unsweetened peanut butter

2 tablespoons coconut aminos

1 teaspoon garlic powder

1 teaspoon ginger powder

1 teaspoon freshly squeezed lime juice

½ teaspoon chili garlic sauce

¼ teaspoon salt

1. Add the tofu, peanut butter, coconut aminos, garlic powder, ginger powder, lime juice, chili garlic sauce, and salt to a blender.

2. Blend on low for about 30 to 60 seconds or until smooth.

STORAGE TIP: Store in an airtight container for up to 7 days for the best freshness.

PER SERVING (3 TABLESPOONS): Calories: 92; Protein: 5g; Fat: 6g; Carbohydrates: 5g; Fiber: 2g; Sugar: 2g; Sodium: 309mg

Serving Recommendations

LIQUID: 1 to 2 tablespoons

PUREE: 2 to 3 tablespoons

SOFT FOODS: 3 tablespoons

GENERAL: 4 tablespoons

Creamy Marinara Dipping Sauce

MAKES ¾ CUP / PREP TIME: 5 MINUTES / COOK TIME: 5 MINUTES

Treats like Almond-Crusted Mozzarella Sticks (page 148) and Cheesy Cauliflower Tots (page 146) taste great alone, but they taste even better with a dipping sauce like a creamy marinara sauce. This simple sauce combines tomato sauce, Parmesan cheese, and Greek yogurt to provide a healthy, protein-rich sauce to pair with your favorite snacks.

½ cup nonfat plain
Greek yogurt

½ cup low-sodium
tomato sauce

2 tablespoons grated
Parmesan cheese

1 teaspoon Italian
seasoning

½ teaspoon garlic powder

¼ teaspoon salt

1. In a small saucepan, combine the yogurt, tomato sauce, Parmesan cheese, Italian seasoning, garlic powder, and salt and heat over medium-low heat.

2. Cook for 3 to 5 minutes, stirring frequently, or until the cheese is melted and the sauce is warmed.

STORAGE TIP: Store in an airtight container in the refrigerator for 1 to 2 weeks.

PER SERVING (3 TABLESPOONS): Calories: 36; Protein: 4g; Fat: 1g; Carbohydrates: 3g; Fiber: 2g; Sugar: 2g; Sodium: 226mg

Serving Recommendations

LIQUID: 2 to 4 tablespoons

PUREE: about ¼ cup

SOFT FOODS: ¼ to ½ cup

GENERAL: about ½ cup

Blue Cheese and Yogurt Dressing

MAKES ABOUT 1¼ CUPS / PREP TIME: 5 MINUTES

Whether with chicken wings, carrot sticks, or over salad, blue cheese dressing can enhance whatever you're eating. This recipe takes the creamy texture and cheesy flavor that you love about blue cheese dressing and recreates them in a lower-fat form. This dressing also tastes great as a drizzle on wraps or a spread on sandwiches. Feel free to add more blue cheese crumbles to the blended dressing for a chunky dressing, but keep in mind that this adds more fat and calories to the recipe and may be difficult to eat for those on a liquid or puree diet.

1 cup nonfat plain
   Greek yogurt

¼ cup crumbled
   blue cheese

1 tablespoon freshly
   squeezed lemon juice

1 teaspoon garlic powder

¼ teaspoon salt

Dash freshly ground
   black pepper

1. Add the yogurt, blue cheese, lemon juice, garlic powder, salt, and pepper to a blender.

2. Blend on medium speed for about 60 seconds, or until smooth.

> **STORAGE TIP:** Store in an airtight container and refrigerate for up to 7 days.

PER SERVING (3 ½ TABLESPOONS): Calories: 50; Protein: 6g; Fat: 2g; Carbohydrates: 2g; Fiber: <0.1g; Sugar: 1g; Sodium: 261mg

Serving Recommendations

LIQUID: 1 to 2 tablespoons

PUREE: 2 to 3 tablespoons

SOFT FOODS: 3 tablespoons

GENERAL: 4 tablespoons

Vegan Cheesy Seasoning Mix

MAKES ABOUT ¼ CUP / PREP TIME: 5 MINUTES

When you can't decide what seasoning you want to use on your food, this all-purpose savory seasoning mix can help. A combination of cheesy flavor along with spice and herbs is reminiscent of nacho chips but could just as easily be sprinkled on a salad, rice dish, or vegetables.

4 tablespoons
    nutritional yeast

1 teaspoon fresh or dried
    dillweed

1 teaspoon garlic powder

1 teaspoon chili
    pepper powder

¼ teaspoon salt

Dash freshly ground
    black pepper

Serving Recommendations

PUREE: 1 to 2 teaspoons

SOFT FOODS: about
1 tablespoon (3 teaspoons)

GENERAL: about
2 tablespoons, or as tolerated

In a small bowl, combine the nutritional yeast, dillweed, garlic powder, chili pepper powder, salt, and pepper.

STORAGE TIP: Store in a tightly sealed container at room temperature in a cool, dry area such as a spice rack or pantry cabinet. Consume within 1 year for best freshness.

PER SERVING (3 TEASPOONS): Calories: 17; Protein: 2g; Fat: 0g; Carbohydrates: 2g; Fiber: 1g; Sugar: 0g; Sodium: 98mg

Vegetable Dill Dip

MAKES ¾ CUP / PREP TIME: 5 MINUTES

Vegetables can provide a healthier crunchy alternative to salty snacks. However, you may miss the dip that usually goes along with chips. This yogurt-based vegetable dip has a refreshing, yet savory, flavor that pairs well with not only vegetables, but also can act as a dip for your favorite protein or a spread for a wrap.

1 cup nonfat plain
  Greek yogurt

½ cup chopped
  broccoli florets

1 teaspoon dried or fresh
  dillweed

1 teaspoon garlic powder

¼ teaspoon ground
  turmeric

¼ teaspoon salt

1. Add the yogurt, broccoli, dillweed, garlic powder, turmeric, and salt to a blender.

2. Blend on high speed for about 1 to 2 minutes, until smooth.

STORAGE TIP: Store in an airtight container in the refrigerator for up to 7 days for best freshness.

PER SERVING (3 TABLESPOONS): Calories: 27; Protein: 5g; Fat: 0g; Carbohydrates: 3g; Fiber: 1g; Sugar: 2g; Sodium: 166mg

Serving Recommendations
LIQUID: 1 to 2 tablespoons
PUREE: 2 to 3 tablespoons
SOFT FOODS: 3 tablespoons
GENERAL: 4 tablespoons, or more as tolerated

Low-Carb Honey Mustard Yogurt Dressing

MAKES ABOUT 1 CUP / PREP TIME: 5 MINUTES

There's nothing like sweet honey mustard drizzled over chicken tenders. This re-creation of the tasty sauce allows you to enjoy the flavor with less sugar and in the creamy form of a salad dressing you can enjoy over salads, meats, or wraps. If you enjoy a sweeter taste, feel free to add a bit more honey, but remember you'll also be adding a bit more carbohydrates, too.

1 cup nonfat plain Greek yogurt

4 teaspoons yellow mustard

1 teaspoon honey

1 teaspoon stevia or no-calorie sweetener

¼ teaspoon salt

1. Add the yogurt, mustard, honey, stevia, and salt to a blender.

2. Blend on low for about 30 seconds or until well-incorporated.

STORAGE TIP: Store in an airtight container in the refrigerator for up to 7 days.

PER SERVING (3 TABLESPOONS): Calories: 31; Protein: 5g; Fat: <1g; Carbohydrates: 4g; Fiber: <1g; Sugar: 3g; Sodium: 217mg

Serving Recommendations

LIQUID: about 1 tablespoon

PUREE: 1 to 2 tablespoons

SOFT FOODS: 2 to 3 tablespoons

GENERAL: 3 to 4 tablespoons

Heart-Healthy Nutty Salad Topper

MAKES ½ CUP / PREP TIME: 3 MINUTES

When you want to enjoy salad, croutons are often the primary choice of topper. However, if you can't tolerate bread, follow a gluten-free lifestyle, or just want to limit carbohydrates, then croutons are a no-go. That doesn't mean that you can't still enjoy a crunch on your salad. This salad topper contains the top heart-healthy nuts and a dash of salt that can be enjoyed alone or on top of your favorite salad, oatmeal, or yogurt dish.

2 tablespoons chopped raw or roasted walnuts

2 tablespoons roasted slivered almonds

2 tablespoons unsalted roasted pistachios

2 tablespoons unsalted roasted peanuts

1 teaspoon extra-virgin olive oil

Dash salt

Dash freshly ground black pepper *(optional)*

1. In a medium mixing bowl, combine the walnuts, almonds, pistachios, and peanuts.

2. Drizzle the nut mixture with oil and toss to coat evenly.

3. Sprinkle with salt and pepper (if using).

STORAGE TIP: Store in an airtight container in your pantry for 3 to 6 months.

PER SERVING (2 TABLESPOONS): Calories: 85; Protein: 3g; Fat: 8g; Carbohydrates: 3g; Fiber: 1g; Sugar: 1g; Sodium: 50mg

Serving Recommendations
GENERAL: about 2 tablespoons

Low-Fat Creamy Cheddar Cheese Sauce

MAKES 1 CUP / PREP TIME: 5 MINUTES / COOK TIME: 4 MINUTES

Cheese sauce can make just about any food taste better. Unfortunately, cheese sauces you buy in the store or eat at a restaurant are usually high in fat and sodium. However, if you replace the cream with Greek yogurt, you can still enjoy a creamy cheese sauce for your veggies or meats. If you prefer a thicker sauce, reduce the almond milk to ¼ cup.

1 tablespoon unsalted butter

1 tablespoon cornstarch

½ cup unsweetened almond milk

½ cup shredded Cheddar cheese

½ cup nonfat plain Greek yogurt

¼ teaspoon salt

Serving Recommendations

LIQUID: 2 to 4 tablespoons

PUREE: ¼ cup 4 to 6 tablespoons

SOFT FOODS: 6 tablespoons

GENERAL: 6 to 8 tablespoons

1. In a medium skillet, heat the butter over medium heat.

2. As the butter melts, stir in the cornstarch with a wooden spoon. Add the almond milk and mix well.

3. Bring to a rolling boil, 1 to 2 minutes, then reduce to a simmer.

4. Mix in the Cheddar cheese and yogurt, a few tablespoons of each at a time, stirring constantly, until all the cheese has been added and is melted into a smooth sauce.

5. Simmer for 1 to 2 minutes while adding in salt and mixing well. Enjoy.

STORAGE TIP: Try to use the sauce upon cooking for maximum freshness, but it can be refrigerated in an airtight container for up to 7 days.

PER SERVING (4 TABLESPOONS): Calories: 103; Protein: 6g; Fat: 8g; Carbohydrates: 3g; Fiber: <1g; Sugar: 1g; Sodium: 258mg

MEASUREMENT CONVERSIONS

VOLUME EQUIVALENTS	U.S. STANDARD	U.S. STANDARD (OUNCES)	METRIC (APPROXIMATE)
LIQUID	2 tablespoons	1 fl. oz.	30 mL
	¼ cup	2 fl. oz.	60 mL
	½ cup	4 fl. oz.	120 mL
	1 cup	8 fl. oz.	240 mL
	1½ cups	12 fl. oz.	355 mL
	2 cups or 1 pint	16 fl. oz.	475 mL
	4 cups or 1 quart	32 fl. oz.	1 L
	1 gallon	128 fl. oz.	4 L
DRY	⅛ teaspoon	—	0.5 mL
	¼ teaspoon	—	1 mL
	½ teaspoon	—	2 mL
	¾ teaspoon	—	4 mL
	1 teaspoon	—	5 mL
	1 tablespoon	—	15 mL
	¼ cup	—	59 mL
	⅓ cup	—	79 mL
	½ cup	—	118 mL
	⅔ cup	—	156 mL
	¾ cup	—	177 mL
	1 cup	—	235 mL
	2 cups or 1 pint	—	475 mL
	3 cups	—	700 mL
	4 cups or 1 quart	—	1 L
	½ gallon	—	2 L
	1 gallon	—	4 L

OVEN TEMPERATURES

FAHRENHEIT	CELSIUS (APPROXIMATE)
250°F	120°C
300°F	150°C
325°F	165°C
350°F	180°C
375°F	190°C
400°F	200°C
425°F	220°C
450°F	230°C

WEIGHT EQUIVALENTS

U.S. STANDARD	METRIC (APPROXIMATE)
½ ounce	15 g
1 ounce	30 g
2 ounces	60 g
4 ounces	115 g
8 ounces	225 g
12 ounces	340 g
16 ounces or 1 pound	455 g

REFERENCES

Alberts, B., A. Johnson, J. Lewis, et al. *Molecular Biology of the Cell, 4th edition.* 2002. New York: Garland Science.

American Society for Metabolic and Bariatric Surgery. "Bariatric Surgery: Postoperative Concerns." Accessed April 18, 2020. https://asmbs.org/resources/bariatric-surgery -postoperative-concerns.

American Society for Metabolic and Bariatric Surgery. "Life After Bariatric Surgery." Accessed February 20, 2020. https://asmbs.org/patients/life-after -bariatric-surgery.

Berrazaga, Insaf, Valérie Micard, Marine Gueugneau, and Stéphane Walrand. "The Role of the Anabolic Properties of Plant- versus Animal-Based Protein Sources in Supporting Muscle Mass Maintenance: A Critical Review." *Nutrients*, 11(8) (2019): 1825. https://doi.org/10.3390/nu11081825.

Carbone, John W., and Stephan M. Pasiakos. "Dietary Protein and Muscle Mass: Translating Science to Application and Health Benefit." *Nutrients,* 11(5) (2019): 1136. doi: 10.3390/nu11051136.

Faria, Silvia Leite, et al. "Recommended Levels of Carbohydrate After Bariatric Surgery." *Bariatric Times*, 10(3) (2013): 16–21.

Gardner, Christopher D., Jennifer C. Hartle, Rachel D. Garrett, Lisa C. Offringa, and Arlin S. Wasserman,. "Maximizing the Intersection of Human Health and the Health of the Environment with Regard to the Amount and Type of Protein Produced and Consumed in the United States." *Nutrition Reviews*, 77(4) (2019): 197–215. https://doi.org/10.1093/nutrit/nuy073.

Johns Hopkins Medicine, Johns Hopkins Bayview Medical Center. "Nutrition Guidelines for Weight Loss Surgery." Accessed April 18, 2020. https://www.hopkinsmedicine .org/johns_hopkins_bayview/_docs/medical_services/bariatrics/nutrition -guidelines-for-weight-loss-surgery.pdf.

Kostecka, Małgorzata, and Monika Bojanowska. "Problems in Bariatric Patient Care— Challenges for Dieticians." *Wideochir Inne Tech Maloinwazyjne,* 12(3) (2017): 207–215. doi: 10.5114/wiitm.2017.70193.

Lonnie, Marta., et al. "Protein for Life: Review of Optimal Protein Intake, Sustainable Dietary Sources and the Effect on Appetite in Ageing Adults." *Nutrients*, 10(3) (2018): 360. https://doi.org/10.3390/nu10030360.

Lupoli, Roberta, et al. "Bariatric Surgery and Long-Term Nutritional Issues." *World Journal of Diabetes*, 8(11) (2017): 464–474. doi: 10.4239/wjd.v8.i11.464.

National Institutes of Health, Office of Dietary Supplements. "Vitamin B12." Accessed April 15, 2020. https://ods.od.nih.gov/factsheets/VitaminB12-HealthProfessional/.

National Sleep Foundation. "A Good Night's Sleep Can Help You Maintain a Healthy Weight." Accessed April 19, 2020. https://www.sleepfoundation.org/excessive -sleepiness/health-impact/good-nights-sleep-can-help-you-maintain -healthy-weight.

Palmer, Sharon. "Vitamin B12 and the Vegan Diet." *Today's Dietitian,* 20(4) (2018): 38. https://www.todaysdietitian.com/newarchives/0418p38.shtml.

Penn Medicine. "What Do You Eat After Bariatric Surgery?" 2019. Accessed April 15, 2020. https://www.pennmedicine.org/updates/blogs/metabolic-and-bariatric -surgery-blog/2019/may/what-you-eat-after-bariatric-surgery.

University of Michigan Medicine. "High-Protein Foods for Wound Healing." Accessed April 15, 2020. https://www.uofmhealth.org/health-library/abs1199.

UCSF Health. "Dietary Guidelines After Bariatric Surgery." Accessed April 19, 2020. https://www.ucsfhealth.org/education/dietary-guidelines-after-bariatric-surgery.

U.S. National Library of Medicine. "What Are Proteins and What Do They Do?" Accessed April 15, 2020. https://ghr.nlm.nih.gov/primer/howgeneswork/protein.

INDEX

ACKNOWLEDGMENTS

Writing and publishing a book has been a goal of mine since middle school. It wasn't until graduate school that I realized my true passion was nutrition and that by using writing and nutrition together I could help people learn to be healthier. I have so many people to thank for helping make this goal a reality.

I want to first thank God for giving me the opportunity to write this book and for blessing me with a pursuit that I enjoy. None of this would be possible without you.

Thank you to my mom and dad, Darlene and Tom McGonigal, as well as my siblings, Tom McGonigal Jr. and Kelly Boyer, for always believing in me and supporting me.

Thank you to my husband, Dennis, for supporting me as I started my writing career from scratch after working as a dietitian full-time. Also, thank you for taste testing all the recipes in this book to make sure they tasted the best they could.

Thank you to my puppy, Ellie, for sitting by my feet as I developed these recipes.

Thank you to my former co-workers and patients at Legacy Weight and Diabetes Institute in Portland, Oregon, for teaching me all about bariatric nutrition and helping me improve my skills as a nutrition counselor.

Thank you to my boss, Karey Schutte at Denver Health, for always believing in my abilities as a dietitian and working with me so I could maintain my job at the hospital while writing this book. And thank you to my Denver Health co-workers for helping me to grow as a dietitian every day.

Thank you to my late grandmother, Louise Bangert, for teaching me just about everything she knew about cooking. Her infamous down-home Southern recipes inspired some of the recipes in this book.

And, finally, a big thank you to my editor, Rachelle Cihonski, as well as Ashley Popp and everyone at Callisto Media for believing in me to write this book and supporting me throughout the writing process.

ABOUT THE AUTHOR

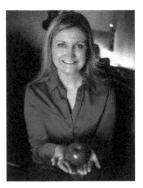

Staci Gulbin, MS, MEd, RD, is a registered dietitian, freelance writer, health editor, and founder of LighttrackNutrition.com. She has been a registered dietitian with the Commission on Dietetic Registration since 2010 and has over a decade of experience in the nutrition and dietetics industry.

Staci has graduate degrees in biology, human nutrition, and nutrition and education from New York University; the Columbia University Institute of Human Nutrition; and Teacher's College, Columbia University, respectively. She has treated thousands of patients across many wellness arenas such as weight management, fitness, long-term care, rehab, and bariatric nutrition.

Since 2011, Staci has been applying her health and wellness knowledge to writing and editing for websites like CDiabetes, Anirva, and Casa de Sante. She has also been featured as an expert in online publications for Shape.com, ThisisInsider.com, Eat This Not That, and more.

Staci hopes her writing and recipes can inspire many to learn to cook and eat healthily so they can expand their palate and create a healthier lifestyle for themselves. She hopes to help make healthy eating seem more accessible, no matter your cooking skill set or budget, and to make healthy food taste delicious so it's something you want to eat all the time.

Printed in the USA
CPSIA information can be obtained
at www.ICGtesting.com
LVHW061532111223
765798LV00007B/22